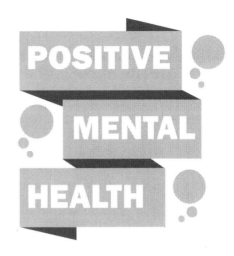

POSITIVE

MENTAL

HEALTH

SOCIAL MEDIA AND MENTAL HEALTH

IN SCHOOLS

WITHDRAWN

POSITIVE MENTAL HEALTH

This new series of texts presents a modern and comprehensive set of evidence-based strategies for promoting positive mental health in schools. There is a growing prevalence of mental ill health among children and young people within a context of funding cuts, strained services and a lack of formal training for teachers. The series recognises the complexity of the issues involved, the vital role that teachers play, and the current education and health policy frameworks in order to provide practical guidance backed up by the latest research.

Our titles are also available in a range of electronic formats. To order, or for details of our bulk discounts, please go to our website www. criticalpublishing.com or contact our distributor, NBN International, 10 Thornbury Road, Plymouth PL6 7PP, telephone 01752 202301 or email orders@nbninternational.com.

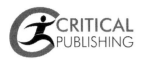

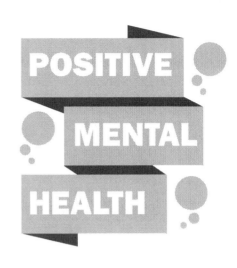

SOCIAL MEDIA AND MENTAL HEALTH

IN SCHOOLS

Jonathan Glazzard and Colin Mitchell

First published in 2018 by Critical Publishing Ltd

The authors have made every effort to ensure the accuracy of information contained in this publication, but assume no responsibility for any errors, inaccuracies, inconsistencies and omissions. Likewise, every effort has been made to contact copyright holders. If any copyright material has been reproduced unwittingly and without permission the publisher will gladly receive information enabling them to rectify any error or omission in subsequent editions.

British Library Cataloguing in Publication Data
A CIP record for this book is available from the British Library

ISBN: 978-1-912508-16-7

This book is also available in the following e-book formats:

MOBI ISBN: 978-1-912508-17-4
EPUB ISBN: 978-1-912508-18-1
Adobe e-book ISBN: 978-1-912508-19-8

Cover and text design by Out of House Limited
Project Management by Out of House Publishing Solutions
Printed and bound in Great Britain by 4edge, Essex

Critical Publishing
3 Connaught Road
St Albans
AL3 5RX

www.criticalpublishing.com

Paper from responsible sources

+ CONTENTS

+MEET THE SERIES EDITOR AND AUTHORS

JONATHAN GLAZZARD

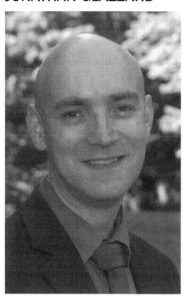

COLIN MITCHELL

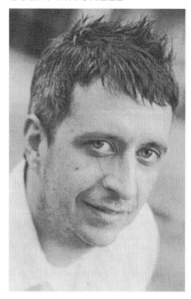

Jonathan Glazzard is series editor for *Positive Mental Health*. He is Professor of Teacher Education at Leeds Beckett University and also the professor attached to the Carnegie Centre of Excellence for Mental Health in Schools. He teaches across a range of QTS and non-QTS programmes and is an experienced teacher educator.

Colin Mitchell has been working with learning technologies in higher education for more than ten years. He is passionate about empowering students and academics to harness technology to enhance teaching and learning. He is also a firm believer that technology is not always the answer and sometimes the best approach can be a simple one.

✛INTRODUCTION

This book addresses the role of social media and its contribution to the mental health of children and young people. It explores the positive and negative effects of social media on mental health and the responsibilities of schools, parents and other stakeholders.

Social media has revolutionised the way in which we interact. Social media use has increased in recent years, and it has become an integral part of children and young people's lives. Internet use has changed dramatically over the past two decades. From originally being a repository of information, the internet has evolved into an essential interactive tool for social collaboration. Increasing forms of connectivity between devices, people and applications are resulting in the creation of a digital universe in the third generation of the world wide web. Teachers need to keep abreast of these developments by embracing the opportunities of more advanced forms of internet-based learning.

We argue that total bans on technology in schools are not helpful because they restrict opportunities for learning. Young people live their lives online and denying them this opportunity is, in effect, cutting off their oxygen supply. However, schools need to be aware of the negative effects of the internet on children and young people. Schools play a key role in providing a digital curriculum which teaches digital citizenship, digital literacy and digital resilience. Digital literacy is the ability to be able to critically evaluate content and learn key skills to stay safe online. Digital citizenship fosters appropriate behaviour online through developing knowledge of acceptable and unacceptable online behaviours and the impact of children and young people's online behaviour on others. Digital resilience relates to knowing how to seek help, and learning from and recovering from negative experiences.

In this book we argue that the way in which young people interact with technology is continuing to change. Everyone has a right to be online and to experience the numerous benefits that this brings. It is everyone's responsibility to ensure that children and young people are protected from harm by reporting and challenging abuse. While it might not be possible to eradicate harmful content from the internet, educating children and young people about their responsibilities as digital citizens and providing them with the skills to enable them to critically evaluate content are appropriate ways of responding to some of the challenges. Fostering young people's digital resilience enables them to bounce back from negative experiences. Schools and parents play an equal role in supporting the development of these skills. The digital industry also plays a significant role in protecting children from harm. Behaviour which is not tolerated offline should also not be tolerated online. Thus, the right of individuals to lead a digital life must be balanced against the extent to which they fulfil their responsibilities as digital citizens to the digital community.

Teachers also need to reflect on their online behaviour. What is posted online stays online and posts from several years earlier can come back to haunt people. Teachers can even lose their careers for posting comments, videos or images which bring their schools into disrepute. As a teacher you have a responsibility to use social media responsibly and to consider the impact that your posts will have now and in the future. While teachers have a right to a private life, parents, children and young people will search for profiles of teachers and, in some cases, they will use these to attempt to destroy careers. We illustrate some of the issues for teachers through case studies.

This book provides valuable insight into the effects of social media on children and young people. We argue that schools and teachers cannot solve the issues in isolation. There is a need for parents, social media companies and children and young people to take responsibility.

We hope that you find this book useful and informative.

Jonathan Glazzard and Colin Mitchell

✚ CHAPTER 1

YOUNG PEOPLE AND TECHNOLOGY

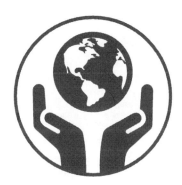

PROFESSIONAL LINKS

This chapter addresses the following:

✍ The national curriculum in computing states that children and young people must be taught to be responsible, competent, confident and creative users of information and communication technology.

CHAPTER OBJECTIVES

By the end of this chapter you will understand:

+ Web 3.0;

+ how children and young people interact with technology;

+ social media use among primary-aged children;

+ social media use among young people in secondary schools.

INTRODUCTION

Young people's use of technology is affected by industry, advertising and the media. All of these stakeholders play a critical role in promoting positive child mental health. This chapter examines young people's use of social media. In addition, it examines the unique contribution that each sector makes to mental health outcomes for children and young people. Key issues are identified, and recommendations are made to support each sector to make a positive contribution to child mental health.

TYPES OF SOCIAL MEDIA PLATFORMS INCLUDING INSTANT MESSAGING PLATFORMS

Children and young people use a variety of platforms in addition to Facebook and Twitter. These include the following.

+ Instagram is a picture and video sharing app. Young people can post content and share experiences, thoughts or memories with an online community. Instagram allows live streaming.

+ Snapchat is an app that enables a user to send a photo, short video or message to their contacts. The 'snap' appears on screen for up to ten seconds before disappearing, or there is an option to have no time limit.

+ YouTube allows users to watch, create and comment on videos. It is possible to create a personal YouTube account, create a music playlist, and even create a personal channel, which requires individuals to have a public profile. YouTube allows live streaming.

+ Minecraft is a game that enables users to build and create a virtual world using building blocks.

+ WhatsApp is an instant messaging app which lets users send messages, images and videos in one-to-one and group chats with their contacts.

This is not an exhaustive list and the variety of platforms will grow as new platforms are introduced. However, these are the common platforms that are used by children and young people.

WEB 3.0 PLATFORMS

Web 1.0 was the first version of the internet. This provided access to websites with information, but users rarely interacted with them. Web 2.0 was a more sophisticated version of the web which enabled users to interact with content and collaborate with each other through a variety of platforms including social media. Web 3.0 is the third generation of internet-based services. It emphasises the following:

+ we live in a digital universe;

+ total connectivity between devices, data, applications and people;

+ devices interact with each other;

+ technology is placed in the hands of students who use it for learning.

In many ways, Web 3.0 is already a reality. We can enable our mobile phones to interact with our cars so that we can speak to people hands-free while we drive. We can control the heating system in our homes via our phones. We can use our mobile phones to view our homes when we are not at home through connecting them with cameras and burglar alarms at home. Data stored in one application can interact with data in another application. We can programme our toaster through our phones. In the future, there will be many more possibilities. Web 3.0 emphasises the complexity of the web and the importance of internet connectivity between devices and applications.

The implications for schools are significant. All schools are engaging in Web 1.0 by providing children and young people with access to the internet. Some schools have not caught up with Web 2.0 because they do not provide learners with opportunities to collaborate and interact via technology. Web 3.0 will present new opportunities for schools but it will involve a culture shift. Schools must keep pace with the changes in technology use in order to ensure that the next generation have the skills they need to operate effectively and efficiently within the twenty-first century. Web 3.0 will result in the internet being available on an increasing range of devices. We already have watches which are internet enabled and there will be an increasing range of devices that will be linked to the internet. Desktop PCs and even laptops will become redundant.

Web 3.0 has implications for schools. This is the vision: everyone will interact with technology to learn and teach. Teachers will teach students, students will teach students and students will teach teachers. Parents will view school as a place for them to learn. Teachers will be everywhere and schools will be everywhere as access to knowledge will not be limited to one place (the school) and the teacher will no longer be the expert.

CRITICAL QUESTIONS

+ Can technology replace the teacher?

+ What other examples of Web 3.0 are currently evident?

+ How will schools use technology in the future?

SOCIAL MEDIA USE: PRIMARY

The *Life in 'Likes'* research found that primary school children use Snapchat, Instagram, Musical.ly and WhatsApp (Children's Commissioner, 2018). This research also found that children accessed their parents' Facebook or Twitter accounts. In primary schools, particularly in Year 4 or below, children may not check their social media accounts frequently. Some children may not have access to technology and may only have access to social media through their parents' devices. However, by Year 5 and 6 most children have access to their own mobile phone. Younger children in primary schools enjoy using technology for entertainment and experimentation purposes. By Year 6, children start using social media as a way of cementing friendships.

Popular platforms include the following.

+ *Roblox is a gaming website and app that enables users to play millions of user-generated games. It is advertised as a 'social platform for play' as users can create groups and message other players.*

+ *Musical.ly is an app that allows you to create and share 15-second videos. Users can choose a song to accompany the video and use photo filters.*

(Children's Commissioner, 2018)

CRITICAL QUESTIONS

+ Most social media platforms have a minimum age limit of 13. Should children in primary schools be allowed to have their own social media accounts?

+ What are the responsibilities of parents in relation to children's use of social media?

+ What are the responsibilities of schools in relation to educating children about social media?

+ Should primary school children have their own mobile phone?

🕑 One in three internet users are children.

🕑 Almost one in four of 8 to 11 year-olds have a social media profile.

🕑 One in four children have experienced something upsetting on a social networking site.

🕑 One in eight children have been bullied on social media.

🕑 Almost one in four children have come across racist or hate messages online.

🕑 Three in four parents have looked for or received information or advice about how to help their child manage online risks.

(www.nspcc.org.uk)

The *Life in 'Likes'* research found the following.

+ Children in Years 4 and 5 were experimenting with a variety of different social media platforms.

+ They had not yet developed habits of checking all their social media on a regular basis.

+ Many, particularly those in Year 4, were accessing social media on their parents' devices, and therefore had limited time to use social media.

+ Children from Years 4–7 used social media to boost their mood and make them laugh, by watching funny videos and sending funny things to their friends.

+ Those in Year 4 were attracted to the games element on certain social media, such as Roblox.

+ In Year 5 social media gave them a platform to be creative and experiment, for example by following baking tutorials.

+ Staying safe online was a priority for many of the younger children.

+ Some felt uncomfortable and bothered when their parents shared some photos of them online.

+ Social media was rarely seen a source of news about the world for children but they saw it as a way of obtaining news about celebrities.

+ Children enjoyed how social media enabled them to be 'in touch' with everyone in their lives.

+ Children in Year 6 identified that it was often hard to interpret the motivation behind comments online, and several cited examples of where they felt something meant as a flippant comment had been misinterpreted.

+ In Year 6 children started to realise that they could change how they looked online and could work out how good other people thought they looked.

(Children's Commissioner, 2018)

CASE STUDY

Sam was in Year 6. He owned his own mobile phone and had developed an interest in several gaming sites. He was allowed to take his phone to bed with him and had started to play games until midnight. As soon as he woke up in the morning he reached for his mobile phone to play games. He wanted to continually improve his scores. He started to avoid going out with his friends, and in the evenings he stayed in his bedroom so that he could play games. He was not allowed to use his phone at school but he did use it to play games the rest of the time. He had stopped communicating with his family during breakfast and dinner times as he interacted with the technology rather than people. On rare occasions, his parents became so frustrated at his lack of communication that they confiscated his mobile phone. During these occasions Sam appeared to be frustrated and depressed.

CRITICAL QUESTIONS

+ Imagine that you are Sam's parent. How would you address the issues?

+ Is Sam's behaviour a concern?

+ What role do schools play in teaching children about the safe and responsible use of technology?

SOCIAL MEDIA USE: SECONDARY

In secondary schools, young people use social media as a way of fitting in and connecting with others. It enables them to keep in touch with friends and not miss out on things that are going on. Some young people use social media as a way of obtaining emotional support from peers. Instagram and Snapchat are popular platforms.

CRITICAL QUESTIONS

+ Some young people are dependent on obtaining likes for things that they have posted online. Is this a good thing?

+ As young people become older, they start to make comparisons between themselves and others they see online. Are there any advantages of doing this? What are the disadvantages?

- One-third of current internet users are under the age of 18.
- Three in four children aged 10–12 have their own social media accounts.

(Children's Commissioner, 2018)

The *Life in 'Likes'* research found the following in the secondary phase of education.

+ Some young people felt concerned that social media could lead to addiction.

+ Young people were constantly contactable and connected, and described this as an important expectation of their friendships.

+ Girls became conscious of how they looked on photos and edited photos to improve their appearance.

+ Young people had started to make comparisons between themselves and others.

+ Both boys and girls felt that many of the things they saw on social media were unattainable to them.

+ As young people grew older, they seemed to care more about the feedback they received on the things they shared on social media.

+ As young people transitioned to secondary school, the desire for peer feedback through likes and comments seemed to become more and more important.

(Children's Commissioner, 2018)

CASE STUDY

Saima was in Year 9. She interacted with a range of social media platforms and regularly uploaded photos and videos to share with others. These uploads enabled Saima to share her experiences with others. She also uploaded several selfies. She had used digital editing software to improve her appearance and had adopted various poses which she had seen celebrities using. Saima had started to monitor how many likes she had received for each of her uploads. If the number of likes was too small she started to become depressed. On several occasions she challenged her friends when they had not acknowledged her posts by asking them why they had not liked them. On a couple of occasions, she ceased her friendships with others when they had not liked her posts.

CRITICAL QUESTIONS

+ Is Saima's behaviour a cause for concern? Explain your response.

+ What support might Saima need?

THE ROLE OF INDUSTRY IN RELATION TO SOCIAL MEDIA

Given the fact that the digital world is now an integral part of young people's lives (Frith, 2017), the digital industry plays an important role in children and young people's mental health. The Internet Safety Strategy (HM Government, 2017a) has emphasised the importance of digital companies adopting the principle of 'think safety first'. Thus, during the development of digital products, safety features should be part of the product design process. These features should include internet safety, cyber security and data protection. Digital companies should build simple reporting mechanisms into their products and response times to complaints should be rapid. Some companies have already introduced walled-garden versions of their digital platforms which are suitable for children; this is an example of good practice which could be rolled out across the digital sector.

Social media and other digital companies have a duty to remove inappropriate content from their platforms rapidly. This includes content which is pornographic, racist, sexist, homophobic, biphobic or transphobic or violent. It also includes inappropriate advertising or live streaming and other content which normalises self-harm, suicide and eating disorders. Digital companies also need to react more rapidly to cyberbullying by suspending the digital accounts of perpetrators and by reporting abuse immediately.

Digital companies should be aware of content that may result in appearance-based comparisons which may subsequently result in body image concerns (RSPH, 2017). Examples include content which promotes the use of cosmetic surgery. Digital companies have a responsibility to add warnings to this content so that children and young people are informed of the associated dangers. Digital companies also have a responsibility to inform young people about the dangers of not respecting their bodies.

The online dating industry has an important responsibility to review processes for ensuring that the user base is over the age of consent. Accounts which belong to people under the age of consent should be terminated. These companies also have a responsibility to report cases where those over the age of sexual consent communicate with those under the age of consent.

The sport industry has already promoted the positive impact that physical activity can have on mental health using various digital platforms. However, it also has a responsibility to highlight the link between body image and mental health needs such as depression, anxiety and eating disorders. Similarly, the beauty industry also has a responsibility to highlight the risks of cosmetic surgery to children and young people via digital platforms. Idealised images which dominate the global beauty industry tend to emphasise fair skin and straight hair (British Youth Council, 2017), which can result in issues of body confidence. Both sectors should use social media to demonstrate their commitment to diverse bodies.

The health sector is experienced in providing specialist support to children and young people with the most serious mental health needs. It plays a crucial role in educating children and young people about mental health and well-being, including physical and social well-being. The health sector has a responsibility to communicate clear information to children and young people using social media. Many young people with mental health needs will turn to social media for support. Charities which support mental health also have a responsibility to provide clear information and guidance to young people through a variety of social media platforms.

THE ROLE OF ADVERTISING IN RELATION TO SOCIAL MEDIA

The Advertising Standards Authority is the regulatory body for the advertising industry. The advertising industry plays a critical role in promoting body positivity. However, research indicates that advertisements in magazines, in newspapers and on social media often portray body confidence in relation to idealised images of beauty (Frith, 2017). Females are often depicted through images of slender bodies which are used to represent beauty and perfection (Frith, 2017). These images and messages can result in young girls and women developing low body confidence, which research suggests can lead to depression, anxiety and the development of eating disorders (British Youth Council, 2017; Frith, 2017). Images and messages about slender, perfect bodies are internalised and this can lead to children and young people developing unrealistic expectations about their own bodies.

While the research suggests that females may be more prone to poor body image than males, it is important to acknowledge that boys and young men can also be affected (British Youth Council, 2017). Advertisements which portray the perfect male body often depict muscular strength as a characteristic of the ideal male body. Research suggests that this can result in males developing an obsession with muscle building, and as a result developing body dissatisfaction (British Youth Council, 2017).

Research also suggests that young people from minority groups may also be affected by body dissatisfaction, for example, young people who identify as lesbian, gay, bisexual or transgender (LGBT). Young people who identify as LGBT may be discriminated against for not conforming to the gendered body expectations of the cisgender majority (British Youth Council, 2017) and this can result in low body esteem. Social media plays a critical role in promoting body confidence.

Research indicates that body dissatisfaction can lead to the development of risky behaviours, which may include smoking, drug, steroid and alcohol use, and either over exercising or not exercising enough (British Youth Council, 2017). Body dissatisfaction can have a negative impact on relationships, education and wider life outcomes (British Youth Council, 2017).

The Advertising Standards Authority has a critical role to play in challenging adverts (including those on social media) which perpetuate stereotypes through depictions of idealised images of gendered bodies. The Authority also has a crucial role to play in ensuring that images of diverse bodies are represented which reflect people's everyday lived experiences in society. This includes ensuring that bodies of people representing minority groups (for example, disability, sexuality, race, ethnicity, non-gender conforming) are represented equally in relation to non-minority groups. The Advertising Standards Authority should also challenge assumptions in adverts that slender or muscular bodies are ideal body types.

THE ROLE OF THE MEDIA IN RELATION TO SOCIAL MEDIA

The media has a responsibility to highlight key issues in relation to child and adolescent mental health through its various channels of communication, including social media. The power of the media lies in the reach of its audience, and the increasing variety of media platforms means that information can be disseminated efficiently to children, young people, parents and educators.

In targeting children and young people, the media can play a key role in their understanding of mental health. The media can play a role in educating young people about how to look after their social, physical and mental health. It can highlight the fact that mental health can fluctuate over time, that poor mental health is not a permanent state and that there are steps they can take to improve their mental health. The media can also play a critical role in signposting children and young people to sources of support. Through television, radio, magazines, newspapers and social media platforms, the media can play an important role in developing mental health literacy and young people can be exposed to the experiences of other young people with mental health needs.

The way in which children and young people interact with the media has changed over time because of the growth of technology. Research suggests that technology is now an integral part of young people's lives and that over a third of those aged 15 in the UK are extreme internet users (Frith, 2017). Media platforms can play a significant role in highlighting to children and young people both the positive and negative impacts of internet use (including social media) on their lives. For example, children and young people need to understand the negative relationship between social media use and life satisfaction (OECD, 2016) and the relationship between social media use, sleep quality and sleep deprivation (Scott et al, 2016). The media has a role to play in highlighting cyberbullying and it can provide advice to children and young people on how to respond to it. In addition, given the normalisation of self-harm and suicide through the introduction of live streaming and sites which normalise eating disorders, the media has a duty of care to highlight the dangers of these to young people.

Media platforms play a critical role in educating children and young people about their responsibilities as digital citizens to the digital community. Through its various platforms the media can support the development of young people's digital literacy and digital resilience skills so that the effects of exposure to harmful content are minimised. Crucially, children and young people need to keep themselves safe online. The media can play an important role in educating young people about the dangers of sexting, grooming and sharing too much personal information with others. In addition, the media has a critical role to play in promoting body confidence through promoting images of diverse bodies and challenging stereotypes of slender and muscular gendered bodies.

The media can play an important role in developing parents' and educators' mental health literacy. It can highlight warning signs, provide information on strategies for supporting children and young people with mental health needs and provide signposting for further information and advice.

SUMMARY

Many children in primary schools have a social media profile and by the end of primary school most children own their own technology. Children initially use social media for entertainment and experimentation purposes. As they get older young people start to use social media as a way of staying connected with their friends and keeping abreast of events which have taken place or are evolving. As children get older they start to make social comparisons between themselves and others on social media and this can result in the development of some mental health needs. The internet has developed from a knowledge repository to a collaborative tool which enables social interaction and collaboration. It will continue to evolve and become increasingly complex as the connectivity between devices, applications and platforms increases, and schools will need to keep abreast of these changes. Social media companies, health and beauty companies, advertising companies and charities all play a critical role in keeping children safe online. Parents and schools also play a key role and this will be addressed in subsequent chapters. In particular, the following points are noted.

+ The digital industry should build safety features into all products which are designed for children and young people as part of the design process. Additionally, it should react more quickly to abuse by removing the accounts of perpetrators and reporting the abuse. It should remove inappropriate content rapidly.

+ The advertising industry should ensure that advertisements, including those on social media platforms, do not promote low body esteem.

+ Media, health and third sector industries all play a crucial role in developing children and young people's mental health literacy via social media platforms and highlighting issues in relation to the mental health of children and young people.

CHECKLIST

This chapter has addressed:

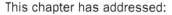 the range of social media platforms which children and young people use;

✓ the purposes for which they use these platforms;

✓ the responsibilities of key stakeholders in relation to social media use.

FURTHER READING

Edgington, S M (2011) *The Parent's Guide to Texting, Facebook, and Social Media: Understanding the Benefits and Dangers of Parenting in a Digital World.* Dallas, TX: Brown Books Publishing Group.

Twenge, J M (2017) *iGen: Why Today's Super-Connected Kids Are Growing Up Less Rebellious, More Tolerant, Less Happy – and Completely Unprepared for Adulthood – and What That Means for the Rest of Us.* New York: Atria Books.

✛ CHAPTER 2

THE BENEFITS
OF SOCIAL MEDIA

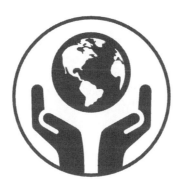

PROFESSIONAL LINKS

This chapter addresses the following:

The national curriculum in computing states that children and young people must be taught to be responsible, competent, confident and creative users of information and communication technology.

CHAPTER OBJECTIVES

By the end of this chapter you will understand:

+ the academic benefits of social media;

+ the social benefits of social media;

+ the psychological benefits of social media.

INTRODUCTION

Young people use social media and the internet for a variety of purposes including forming social connections, looking for support with homework and seeking advice (Frith, 2017). Evidence suggests that young people with mental health problems often turn to social media and the internet for support and advice (Frith, 2017). While the negative impacts are well documented (Frith, 2017; RSPH, 2017), it is important to remember the power of the internet and social media to enrich people's lives. Through various platforms young people can access a wealth of resources and communication opportunities, which would otherwise be restricted due to financial, geographical, social and cultural constraints. Young people who withdraw themselves from the online world due to negative experiences limit themselves from enriching opportunities which can support their academic, social, cultural, political and identity development. Social media can act as an effective platform for positive self-expression, allowing young people to project a positive identity (RSPH, 2017). In addition, social media allows minority groups such as young people who identify as LGBTQ+ to connect with each other and build a sense of community, despite geographical separation (Russel and Fish, 2016). There is also evidence to suggest that strong friendships can be enhanced through social media interaction (Lenhart, 2015).

ACADEMIC BENEFITS

Social media can support academic development through facilitating collaboration and access to information. Boyd (2008) highlights the value of collaborating on projects through online communities, for example, a homework group for people in the same class or closed group for students who are studying for an examination. This can also facilitate interaction with teachers online. Ito et al (2008) highlight the power of social media for sharing new creative projects such as online videos, blogs and podcasts.

The internet has fundamentally changed how young people learn. Prior to the internet, young people were largely dependent on teachers for knowledge. Now knowledge can be accessed almost anywhere. Young people can research subject-specific knowledge online and they can collaborate with others to aid their understanding of knowledge. Teachers therefore need to consider how they are building on the knowledge that is already available in the public domain by supporting learners to apply, synthesise and create knowledge.

Children and young people can access subject-specific information online. If they do not understand a subject-specific concept, they can watch a video on YouTube which clearly explains that concept. They can use online information to create presentations and can search for diagrams, photographs, video and audio information to support subject-specific learning.

Despite these benefits it is important that children and young people can critically evaluate the information that they access online. There is a lot of information on the internet and not all of it is accurate. Schools need to give children the skills to identify which sources are reliable and those which are not. In addition, they need to be able to differentiate between factually accurate information and opinion.

Younger children will benefit from a more focused approach to searching for information. They will find it more manageable to be directed to specific applications and you can scaffold their research by providing them with specific questions to answer.

CRITICAL QUESTIONS

+ How can social media impact on knowledge development?

+ How can social media impact on skills development?

+ How can social media impact on the development of attitudes and values?

19

The 2017 statistics for young people aged 12–15 show that:

- 74 per cent used Facebook;
- 58 per cent used Snapchat;
- 57 per cent used Instagram;
- 32 per cent used YouTube;
- 32 per cent used WhatsApp;
- 19 per cent used Twitter;
- 10 per cent used Musical.ly;
- 7 per cent used Pinterest.

(www.statista.com)

According to *Life in 'Likes'*, social media use had a range of academic benefits.

+ It allowed children to be creative.

+ Social media enabled them to learn new things that would let them achieve their goals.

(Children's Commissioner, 2018)

According to Young Minds:

Young people use social media and online communities as an important distraction from the pressures of studying for exams, a solace from the strains of a challenging family life and to secure instant access to a like-minded community of peers who share their interests, passions and desires... Similarly, when they face a challenging life experience, traumatic event or an episode of poor mental health, they frequently turn to social media platforms... Some children turn to their online friends and communities when they are in distress.

(Young Minds, 2016, p 6)

CASE STUDY

A primary school developed a scheme of peer digital ambassadors. Children were identified who had well-developed digital skills. They were trained in some simple pedagogical approaches and subsequently ran a series of workshops with younger children to help them to develop their digital skills. They introduced the younger children to a variety of applications, including games, and taught them simple digital literacy skills. The sessions were extremely popular. They ran after school as an extra-curricular club and were over-subscribed. The digital peer mentors were also matched with individuals whose computing skills were less well developed. They provided them with informal support during lunchtimes to improve their digital skills.

CRITICAL QUESTIONS

+ What are the benefits of peer mentoring to the mentor?
+ What are the limitations?

SOCIAL BENEFITS THROUGH ONLINE COMMUNITIES

Frith (2017) and Ito et al (2008) highlight how social media enables young people to connect with friends and family, particularly over long distances, by sharing pictures and videos, and therefore addressing social isolation and loneliness. Lenhart et al (2015) have emphasised the role of social media in making new friends, particularly with people with shared interests. Ito et al (2008) discuss the value of social media in facilitating community and political involvement through the formation of networks who come together with a common interest. Use of social media has been associated with improved social skills among adolescents (Rosen, 2011). It can help socially introverted people to become more socially active. Lilley et al (2014) highlight the positive benefits of social media in facilitating young people talking to friends online, developing a vehicle for self-expression and providing children and young people with the opportunity to be creative.

CRITICAL QUESTIONS

+ What are the benefits of connecting with people online?

+ Are online friends just as important as real friends?

In the PISA (2015) well-being study of young people aged 15, 90.5 per cent of boys and 92.3 per cent of girls in the UK agreed or strongly agreed with the statement *'It is very useful to have social networks on the internet'*.

An estimated one in three of all internet users in the world today are below the age of 18.

Four in five of young adults aged between 16 and 24 years believe that digital technology plays a positive role in their relationships.

Around half found online interactions more straightforward than those taking place face to face.

(Young Minds, 2016)

According to *Life in 'Likes'*, social media use had a range of social benefits.

+ Children used social media as a tool to maintain friendships.

+ Children were able to judge the strength of their friendships on social media based on the number of replies they received.

+ Social media allowed them to keep in touch and 'stay in the loop'.

However, the following detrimental effects were identified.

+ Social relationships got more difficult to manage at secondary school, where friendships could break down online.

+ Maintaining online friendships could be stressful for some as they experienced the need to reply to messages immediately.

+ Being offline was viewed as socially damaging for friendships.

(Children's Commissioner, 2018)

IDENTITY DEVELOPMENT

Young people can use a variety of online platforms to explore their identity. This is particularly valuable for those who live in isolated rural communities where there may be fewer opportunities for identity development. They can join online networks and become part of an online community. Through participation in digital communities, young people can explore their interests and develop aspirations. They can communicate with online peers and through this collaboration can form their own views and values.

DEVELOPING AUTONOMY

Young people can develop autonomy through their participation in the digital world. The online world is a space where they can interact freely with others away from the watchful gaze of their parents. While this is advantageous, it is also risky and therefore young people need to be alerted to the dangers of online interactions. They should be taught to keep themselves safe by using privacy settings, and should be taught to block users and to report abuse. It is also important to highlight the dangers associated with the 'dark web'. These are websites which promote self-harm and eating disorders and do not have the same safety functions that are embedded in other websites.

It is important that young people are trusted to use the internet responsibly. Banning them from using the internet will have a detrimental effect because they will resent it. In addition, banning them from using the internet restricts their autonomy, and this is vital during adolescence. Most children and young people will use the internet responsibly if they are trusted to do so, have been taught how to use it responsibly and are aware of the risks.

CASE STUDY

A secondary school developed a closed Facebook group for students who were new to English. Many of these young people were refugees who had recently arrived in the United Kingdom. However, others had been in the country for several years. The group was managed by a group of digital champions whose first language was not English. The young people were able to use the site for a variety of purposes, including sharing information and experiences. Some used it as a source of support. The students found the site valuable as it facilitated the development of an online community of students whose first language was not English. It helped to facilitate a sense of belonging within the school and validated their identities.

CRITICAL QUESTIONS

+ Are there any limitations associated with forming closed online communities?
+ What other digital strategies can be used to facilitate the inclusion of specific groups of students?

PSYCHOLOGICAL BENEFITS

Social media can support identity development during childhood and adolescence. Children and young people can use social media to explore their interests and through interactions with others online can start to develop specific aspirations for their futures. Young people may use social media to access health information online or may form networks with others who are experiencing or have experienced the same health conditions. However, this can be risky because information online may not be factually accurate. Therefore, it is essential that schools teach young people to evaluate online information critically.

O'Keeffe and Clarke-Pearson (2011) have emphasised the role of social media in providing young people with networks that can provide emotional support and advice. Young people at risk of suicide are likely to turn to the internet for support (Frith, 2017). Research suggests that online suicide prevention may be effective, and that social media provides an opportunity to identify problems early and support those at risk (Christensen et al, 2014).

There is evidence that young people turn to online friends when they need support and advice (Young Minds, 2016). They find it particularly useful to communicate with peers who have had similar experiences. This provides them with a wider support network and fosters a sense of community spirit in the digital world. Young people find it useful to turn to online peers when they are feeling distressed.

Children and young people can become more motivated through using social media. Designing tasks which require young people to use social media can therefore increase motivation in lessons.

Social media can also support the development of self-concept and self-esteem. The self-concept (how we view ourselves) is affected by peers, teachers, parents and others. Positive interactions on social media with peers can help young people to develop a positive self-concept. The ideal self (what we aspire to be) can also be enhanced through using social media. Young people have access to role models online. These are people who they aspire to be like. This can have both a positive and negative impact on self-esteem.

Social media can improve social confidence, particularly for those individuals who find it difficult to communicate with others face to face. Through social media some people can 'find their voice'. They become more confident in expressing their views, engaging in online discussions and even develop the confidence to constructively challenge others. Once they are confident in communicating online they can gradually transfer this confidence to offline interactions.

Through participation in the digital world, young people can become more resilient when they experience adversity. During distressing and difficult experiences, they can gain support from online peers and online digital communities and these networks can help to build resilience. Young people may seek support from others if they receive bad news and this can help them to become more resilient.

Social media use can also support intellectual development by providing young people with opportunities to stimulate their minds. Playing online games can support the development of problem-solving skills and improve skills in resilience, planning, prediction and logic. Access to social media can facilitate access to knowledge, which will improve intelligence.

CRITICAL QUESTIONS

+ Is it better to gain emotional support online or face to face?

+ How does social media impact on intellectual development?

+ How might social media impact on personality development?

According to *Life in 'Likes'*, social media use had a range of psychological benefits.

+ Social media made children happy: children knew how to cheer themselves up or calm themselves down using social media.

+ Children tended to associate social media with positive moods and happy emotions.

+ Children felt good when they got likes and comments from friends.

+ Social media use took their mind off things.

+ Young people could gain emotional support from friends.

+ It gave them motivation to aspire to be like others, including role models.

+ Some children developed new aspirations about what they wanted their future to be like.

However, the following detrimental effects were noted.

+ Children were conscious of keeping up appearances on social media; girls were worried about looking 'pretty' and boys were more concerned with looking 'cool' and having the right clothing.

+ Many became aware of how they looked compared to other people on social media and felt that comparisons were unattainable.

(Children's Commissioner, 2018)

 Of the young people contacting Childline, 78 per cent now do so online, via email or online chat, and more counselling from the service (59 per cent) now takes place online than by telephone.

(cited in Frith, 2017)

Half of 9–16 year-olds in Europe now own a smartphone.

Two-thirds of 9–16 year-olds have at least one social media or networking account.

(Young Minds, 2016)

SUMMARY

This chapter has highlighted some of the benefits of social media. The research indicates that social media is now an integral part of young people's lives and that it provides them with a valuable source of social and emotional support. However, it is important to weigh up the benefits against the limitations. We have touched on these in this chapter and devoted a full chapter in this book to the negative impacts of social media. Schools and parents play a critical role in helping children to avoid the detrimental effects and in enabling them to manage these when they encounter adverse experiences online.

CHECKLIST

This chapter has addressed that:

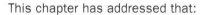 being online makes children and young people happy;

✓ social media enables young people to develop and test friendships;

✓ social media enables young people to learn new skills;

✓ social media facilitates aspiration;

✓ young people use social media as a form of social and emotional support.

FURTHER READING

Puccico, D and Havey, A (2016) *Sex, Likes and Social Media: Talking to Our Teens in the Digital Age*. London: Vermilion.

✛ CHAPTER 3

THE IMPACT OF TECHNOLOGY ON CHILDREN'S WELL-BEING

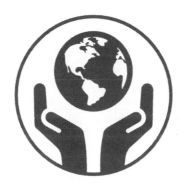

PROFESSIONAL LINKS

This chapter addresses the following:

⬭ The Teachers' Standards emphasise the duty of teachers to safeguard children and young people from risk of harm.

⬭ The national curriculum programmes of study emphasise the role of schools in teaching children and young people to use technology safely, respectfully and responsibly.

CHAPTER OBJECTIVES

By the end of this chapter you will understand:

+ the impact of technology, and specifically social media, on children's well-being;

+ the responsibilities of key stakeholders.

INTRODUCTION

This chapter considers the impact of social media on young people's mental health. It addresses both the positive and negative impacts of social media on young people's lives. In addition, it considers the responsibilities of social media companies, schools and parents in promoting the skills of digital literacy, digital citizenship, digital resilience and minimising exposure to harmful content.

THE CURRENT CONTEXT

According to the Office for National Statistics (ONS) (2016), the proportion of people using the internet daily rose from 35 per cent in 2006 to 82 per cent in 2016 and the use of social media has risen broadly in line with internet use. Social media has revolutionised the way in which we interact, and it has become an integral part of young people's lives (Royal Society for Public Health [RSPH], 2017). Many young people are digital natives; they have never known a world without instant access to the internet. While this presents exciting opportunities for academic, social and identity development, nevertheless, it is a concern that social media has been described as more addictive than cigarettes and alcohol (Hofmann et al, 2012) and it is also worrying that an increasing number of young people experience anxiety and nervousness when they are offline (Frith, 2017).

The 16–24 age group are the most active social media users with 91 per cent using the internet for social media (ONS, 2016). Facebook is the most common platform, followed by Google+, LinkedIn, Pinterest, Instagram and Snapchat (RSPH, 2017). More than a third (37.3 per cent) of young people aged 15 in the UK are classified as 'extreme internet users'. This is defined by the OECD as a young person who uses the internet for more than six hours outside of school on a typical weekend day (cited in Frith, 2017). Evidence suggests that an overwhelming majority (94.8 per cent) of young people aged 15 in the UK used social media before and after school in 2015 (OECD, 2016).

Research indicates that young people's online activity is becoming increasingly private (Frith, 2017). It is conducted in their own bedrooms or via a personal smartphone, thus making it more difficult for parents to monitor their children's online activity. Instant messaging via social media platforms has grown in popularity among young people (Frith, 2017) and this has also made it increasingly difficult for parents to monitor online activity. While this may be a cause for concern, consideration should be given to the benefits of social media use for young people.

THE BENEFITS OF SOCIAL MEDIA AND INTERNET USE

Young people use social media and the internet for a variety of purposes, including forming social connections, seeking support with homework and seeking advice (Frith, 2017). Evidence suggests that young people with mental health problems often turn to social media and the internet for support and advice (Frith, 2017). While the negative impacts are well documented (Frith, 2017; RSPH, 2017), it is important to remember the power of the internet and social media to enrich people's lives. Through various platforms young people can access a wealth of resources and communication opportunities which would otherwise be restricted due to financial, geographical, social and cultural constraints. Young people who withdraw themselves from the online world due to negative experiences limit themselves from enriching opportunities which can support their academic, social, cultural, political and identity development. Social media can act as an effective platform for positive self-expression, allowing young people to project a positive identity (RSPH, 2017). In addition, social media allows minority groups such as young people who identify as LGBTQ+ to connect with each other and build a sense of community, despite geographical separation (Russel and Fish, 2016). There is also evidence to suggest that strong friendships can be enhanced through social media interaction (Lenhart, 2015).

THE NEGATIVE IMPACTS OF SOCIAL MEDIA

Research suggests that excessive internet use can have a detrimental impact on life satisfaction (OECD, 2016). The Office for National Statistics has also found an association between longer time spent on social media and mental health problems; 27 per cent of young people who engage with social networking sites for three or more hours per day experience symptoms of mental ill health compared to 12 per cent of children who spend no time on social networking sites (ONS, 2015). Research suggests that young people who are heavy users of social media are more likely to report poor mental health, including psychological distress (cited in RSPH, 2017). Seeing other people online leading idealised lives can result in unhelpful comparisons, which can result in feelings of inadequacy, anxiety, self-consciousness, low self-esteem and the pursuit of perfectionism (RSPH, 2017).

- 82 per cent of people used the internet on a daily basis in 2016.
- Facebook has 30 million UK users.
- 91 per cent of those aged 16–24 use social media compared with 51 per cent of those aged 55–64 and 23 per cent of the 65-plus age range.

(RSPH, 2017)

SOCIAL MEDIA, ANXIETY AND DEPRESSION

Research suggests that young people who use social media heavily are more likely to report poor mental health, including psychological distress (Sampasa-Kanyinga and Rosamund, 2015). Young people generally post positive messages and images of their lives on social media. These represent idealised lives. Others then begin to make social comparisons between their own lives and the lives of their peers. If they begin to feel that their own life is dull in comparison with that of their peers, this can result in the development of mental health disorders.

- One in six young people will experience an anxiety disorder at some point in their lives.

- Rates of anxiety and depression in young people have increased by 70 per cent over the past 25 years.

- Young people have acknowledged that four of the five most used social media platforms actually make their feelings of anxiety worse.

- 80,000 children and young people in the UK suffer with severe depression.

(RSPH, 2017)

CRITICAL QUESTIONS

+ Why do you think that people tend to represent idealised lives on social media?

+ How can schools educate children and young people about this issue?

SOCIAL MEDIA, SELF-HARM AND SUICIDE

The growth of websites which normalise self-harm and eating disorders promotes unhealthy behaviour. Additionally, the popularity of websites which live stream distressing content, including the live streaming of suicide, is particularly worrying. Self-harm can lead to suicide so it is particularly important that this issue is addressed by schools, parents and external agencies using a co-ordinated approach.

A relationship between internet use and self-harm/suicidal behaviour was particularly associated with internet addiction, high levels of internet use, and websites with self-harm or suicide content.

(Marchant et al, 2018)

Researchers from the University of Manchester found that for girls, the rate of self-harm was 37.4 per 10,000, much higher than 12.3 per 10,000 in boys. It rose by 68 per cent in girls aged 13 to 16 from 45.9 per 10,000 in 2011 to 77.0 per 10,000 in 2014.

(www.manchester.ac.uk/discover/news/steep-rise-in-self-harm-among-teenage-girls)

CRITICAL QUESTIONS

+ What are the responsibilities of social media companies in relation to the live streaming of inappropriate content?

+ Why are girls more likely to self-harm than boys?

+ Why do you think that rates of self-harm have increased?

+ Should all cases of self-harm be referred to child and adolescent mental health services?

SOCIAL MEDIA AND SLEEP DEPRIVATION

There is an association between sleep and mental health. Poor mental health can lead to poor sleep quality and poor sleep quality can lead to poor mental health (cited in RSPH, 2017). Several studies have shown that increased social media use is significantly associated with poor sleep quality in young people (Scott et al, 2016). Using social media on phones, laptops and tablets at night before going to sleep is also linked with poor sleep quality (Woods and Scott, 2016; Xanidid and Brignell, 2016). This can have a detrimental effect on young people's engagement in lessons, and can then impact negatively on their academic progress.

 Adolescents need around one to two hours more sleep every night than adults.

20 per cent of young people wake up during the night to check messages on social media.

(RSPH, 2017)

CRITICAL QUESTIONS

+ What are the responsibilities of parents in relation to this issue?

+ How does sleep quality impact on children's engagement in lessons?

SOCIAL MEDIA AND BODY IMAGE

There is a paucity of research on the impact of social media on young people's body esteem. Research has shown that when young females in their teens and early twenties view Facebook for only a short period of time, body image concerns are higher compared to non-users (Tiggeman and Slater, 2013). The popularity of selfies, the abundance of photoshopped images of celebrities and the prevalence of beautiful bodies can result in lower body esteem and body surveillance (Frith, 2017). This can lead to young people wanting to change their appearance by altering their face, hair or skin. The rise in the number of young people opting to have cosmetic surgery is also a concern.

Time spent on the internet was associated with a decrease in body image satisfaction and problematic eating behaviours. The study also found that female adolescents had lower satisfaction in body image than males.

(Natthakarn et al, 2017)

🖊 70 per cent of 18–24 year-olds would consider having cosmetic surgery.

🖊 Nine in ten girls are unhappy with their body.

🖊 10 million new photographs are uploaded to Facebook alone every hour.

(RSPH, 2017)

CRITICAL QUESTIONS

+ What are the responsibilities of advertising companies in relation to body image?
+ How can schools address the issues associated with body image?
+ What are the responsibilities of parents in relation to body image?
+ What are the issues regarding the digital manipulation of images online?

CASE STUDY

Sunita was in Year 5. For her birthday six months ago, she had been given an iPad. She had started to dramatically lose weight, and had complained on several occasions that the food that her parents had given her at home was 'unhealthy' and 'full of fat'. Sunita's teachers had also noticed the weight loss and the lunchtime supervisors had noticed that she was only eating small portions of food at midday. The school decided to call a meeting with her parents. Sunita's parents attended the meeting. They commented that they had noticed that Sunita was viewing photographs and videos of celebrities and models on her iPad. They had checked her search history. Sunita had also taken photographs of her own body and had used digital editing to make her look slimmer.

CRITICAL QUESTIONS

+ Should Sunita have been present in this meeting? Explain your response.
+ What should the school do next?

SOCIAL MEDIA AND CYBERBULLYING

Cyberbullying is bullying which takes place via the use of technology. It includes:

+ posting hurtful/negative comments in response to another person's posts;

+ uploading malicious comments about another person;

+ uploading videos or photographs which might upset another person;

+ sending private messages which are hurtful.

Cyberbullying is a serious problem which takes a variety of forms. Evidence suggests that it is increasing and that it has a negative impact on young people's confidence and self-esteem (Frith, 2017). Victims respond in a variety of ways; younger children are more likely to talk to their parents, while older children may talk to their friends. Young people need to develop the digital skills to protect themselves, such as blocking users or updating their privacy settings.

Childhood bullying can have long-lasting effects which impact on adulthood. Victims of cyberbullying may experience depression, anxiety, self-harm, changes in eating patterns and poor sleep quality (RSPH, 2017).

Cyberbullying differs from traditional face-to-face bullying in the following ways.

+ Victims cannot escape from it in their own homes.

+ The bullying is witnessed by a larger audience.

+ The evidence of the bullying is permanently online.

+ Perpetrators can anonymously hide behind fake profiles.

+ Harmful content can be repeatedly shared so the victim may experience the effects of the bullying multiple times.

+ Perpetrators tend to be braver online than they would be in a face-to-face situation so the extent of the bullying can be greater.

🌜 70 per cent of young people have experienced cyberbullying.

🌜 91 per cent of young people who reported cyberbullying reported that no action was taken as a result.

🌜 37 per cent of young people experience cyberbullying frequently.

(RSPH, 2017)

CASE STUDY

Tom was 14. He had experienced cyberbullying for three years due to being overweight. He had received abusive and threatening text messages and peers had posted hurtful messages about him online. Initially, Tom did not tell anyone about the abuse. However, over time he gradually became increasingly depressed. He had become so anxious about going online that he deleted all of his social media accounts and changed his mobile phone number so that the perpetrators could not contact him. Eventually, Tom told his teachers and his parents and the matter was addressed through using a restorative approach to behaviour. Tom decided that he wanted to help others and he asked his school if he could become a peer ambassador for other young people who were experiencing or had experienced online abuse. A 'drop-in' service was used to enable Tom to informally support others in the same situation.

CRITICAL QUESTIONS

+ What are the responsibilities of social media companies in relation to cyberbullying?

+ What are the responsibilities of schools in relation to cyberbullying?

SOCIAL MEDIA AND FEAR OF MISSING OUT

Fear of missing out (FOMO) is linked to higher levels of social media engagement; thus, the more an individual uses social media, the more likely they are to experience FOMO. Research suggests that FOMO is associated with lower mood and lower life satisfaction (Przybylski et al, 2013).

By uploading text, photographs and videos people can depict to the world that they are leading a very exciting life. This can lead some individuals to believe that their life is less exciting and that they are missing out on all the fun. Additionally, the fear of missing out on content can lead to sleep deprivation and poor sleep quality. Some young people continually check their social media accounts or text messages during the night when they should be sleeping.

Fear of missing out can also result in constantly checking for messages during social events. This can result in people not fully experiencing what they are doing in the moment and it reduces the quality of social connectivity, which is vital for good mental health.

SOCIAL MEDIA AND EXPOSURE TO INAPPROPRIATE CONTENT

Inappropriate content might include:

+ real or simulated violence;

+ sexually explicit content;

+ illegal images of child sexual abuse;

+ content promoting hate based on race, religion or sexual preference;

+ content instructing or promoting crime or violence;

+ content promoting violent extremism;

+ content that advocates unsafe behaviour. This might include extreme dieting, self-harm, suicide or drug taking.

At 11, the majority of children had not seen online pornography (only 28 per cent of 11–12 year-olds).

By 15, children were more likely than not to have seen online pornography (65 per cent of 15–16 year-olds). Almost all of this group (94 per cent) had seen it by age 14.

Boys were more likely to want to copy activity they had seen (44 per cent compared to 29 per cent of girls).

(Martellozzo et al, 2017)

SOCIAL MEDIA AND GAMING

Online gaming sites which expose young people to violent and sexualised content are also a concern. Gaming disorder is identified in the draft 11th Revision of the International Classification of Diseases. It is characterised by:

+ impaired control over gaming;

+ increasing priority given to gaming over other activities to the extent that gaming takes precedence over other interests and daily activities;

+ the continuation or escalation of gaming despite the occurrence of negative consequences.

(World Health Organisation website)

Impairment in participation in personal, family, social or educational activities may also be characteristic of gaming disorder.

● Young people aged 12–15 spent 12.2 hours a week gaming in 2017.

● Children aged 3–4 spent 5.9 hours per week gaming in 2017.

(The Statistics Portal, www.statista.com)

CRITICAL QUESTIONS

+ What are the beneficial impacts of gaming?

+ What are the responsibilities of parents in relation to gaming?

+ What are the responsibilities of software developers in relation to protecting children and young people from risk of harm?

SOCIAL MEDIA AND SOCIAL ISOLATION

Excessive social media use can result in social isolation. This results in children and young people not developing face-to-face social connections. Face-to-face social connections are vital for positive mental health. Some children and young people who struggle to form friendships may develop online connections. However, this further reduces opportunities for the development of real friendships and limits opportunities for engaging in meaningful activities, such as physical activity, which have a positive effect on well-being.

IMPACT OF INTERNET USE AND SOCIAL MEDIA USE ON ACADEMIC ATTAINMENT

The evidence on the impact of the internet on academic attainment is inconclusive. Children can use the internet as a source of knowledge to aid their academic studies. They can communicate with peers if they need academic support. They can research subject-specific content. However, too much time online can result in poor sleep quality, which can impact detrimentally on academic achievement. Social media use can result in the development of mental health disorders, which can also impact detrimentally on academic attainment. The impact of internet use and social media on attainment is dependent on how children use technology, the purposes for which they use it and the length of time they spend online. Negative experiences online can impact detrimentally on academic attainment.

WARNING SIGNS FOR SOCIAL MEDIA OVERLOAD

It is important that teachers and parents are able to recognise the signs of social media overload. These might include the following.

+ Children and young people who are prone to anxiety and depression may use social media to make them feel better.

+ Signs of social isolation.

+ Those with a limited social life or those who infrequently participate in social activities may be addicted to using technology.

+ If children and young people demonstrate signs of stress, anxiety, frustration, anger, or depression when they cannot access technology, this might indicate that they are experiencing withdrawal effects.

+ Those who interact with technology in social situations rather than with people may be experiencing addiction.

+ Those whose first response when they wake up is to reach for technology may be experiencing addiction.

+ If their use of technology is increasing, this might suggest that the child or young person is developing an addiction.

+ Those who feel that they do not 'fit in' at school and have struggled to establish friendships may turn to technology to form online connections.

+ Some children and young people turn to technology rather than people for comfort when they are upset or are experiencing a low mood. This might suggest that they are developing an unhealthy relationship with technology.

+ When the online world becomes more important than the real world, this could suggest that there might be a problem.

+ Some children and young people might use technology secretly in private even if it has been banned from use.

SCHOOL POLICIES ON SOCIAL MEDIA

Schools operate different policies on mobile technology use. Some schools operate total bans on mobile technology by preventing children and young people from bringing the technology to school. Others allow them to bring the technology to use at break times only. Some schools adopt a more relaxed approach by permitting students to place their phones on their desks during lessons.

CRITICAL QUESTIONS

+ What are your views on total bans on mobile technology in school?

+ What approach do you think is best to adopt?

+ How can teachers utilise mobile technology in lessons?

ADDRESSING THE NEGATIVE EFFECTS OF SOCIAL MEDIA

The Internet Safety Strategy (HM Government, 2017a) emphasises the importance of developing the following in young people.

+ Digital literacy: the ability to be able to critically evaluate content and learn key skills to stay safe online.

+ Digital citizenship: knowledge of acceptable and unacceptable online behaviours and the impact of their online behaviour on others.

+ Digital resilience: knowing how to seek help, learning from and recovering from experience.

Schools should provide an age-appropriate curriculum to young people which focuses on developing these skills. All schools should have appropriate filters and monitoring systems to keep children safe online. Schools should respond to all forms of bullying (online and off-line) which take place outside of school in addition to responding to bullying which takes place in school. Schools should also consider the positive impact that peer–peer support can have by developing anti-bullying digital ambassador schemes.

Parents play a critical role in establishing rules (such as setting time limits), monitoring their child's online activity, talking to their child about online safety and installing filters. Restricting access to social media may not be an appropriate solution because this restricts the development of digital skills which children will need to stay safe online. Schools can play an important role in developing parents' knowledge and skills in internet safety so that they are able to provide appropriate support to their child.

The digital industry also plays a critical role in promptly reporting abuse, removing inappropriate content and suspending the social media accounts of perpetrators. App store providers should build in safety features from the outset to prevent children's exposure to harmful content. Interrupting the user's experience in response to inappropriate searches is also one way in which the digital industry can respond.

What is clear is that the way in which young people interact with technology is continuing to change (Frith, 2017). Everyone has a right to be online and to experience the numerous benefits that this brings. It is everyone's responsibility to ensure that children and young people are protected from harm by reporting and challenging abuse. While it might not be possible to eradicate harmful content, educating children and young people about their responsibilities as digital citizens and providing them with the skills to enable them to critically evaluate content are appropriate ways of responding to some of the challenges outlined in this report. Additionally, developing children's digital resilience will help them to bounce back from negative experiences. Schools

43

and parents play an equal role in supporting the development of these skills. The digital industry also plays a significant role in protecting children from harm. Behaviour which is not tolerated offline should also not be tolerated online. Thus, the right of individuals to lead a digital life must be balanced against the extent to which they fulfil their responsibilities as digital citizens to the digital community.

SUMMARY

This chapter has emphasised the impact of social media on children and young people's mental health. Banning the use of social media is unhelpful because when used responsibly it is a valuable source of information and enables young people to network in ways that once were not possible. Schools play an important role in educating children and young people about the safe and responsible use of social media. However, schools cannot address the issues in isolation. Parents, social media and advertising companies also play an important role in keeping children safe online. In addition, software developers also play an essential role in designing products which are safe for young people to use. This chapter has highlighted some of the issues and suggested some possible solutions.

CHECKLIST

This chapter has addressed that:

✓ social media use can result in mental health issues;

✓ schools play a critical role in educating children about the safe and responsible use of social media;

✓ social media companies play a crucial role responding to online abuse;

✓ software designers have a responsibility to keep young people safe online;

✓ parents play a critical role in encouraging the safe use of social media;

✓ advertising companies play a crucial role in mediating the images that they use to advertise products.

FURTHER READING

Edwards, C (2018) *Social Media and Mental Health: Handbook for Parents and Guardians*. Nottingham: Trigger Press Ltd.

✚ CHAPTER 4

CYBERBULLYING

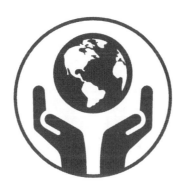

PROFESSIONAL LINKS

This chapter addresses the following:

- The national curriculum for computing requires schools to teach children and young people to use technology safely and responsibly.

- The Teachers' Standards (Part 2) place a professional duty on all teachers to protect children from harm.

CHAPTER OBJECTIVES

By the end of this chapter you will understand:

+ what cyberbullying is and what forms it takes;

+ the effects of cyberbullying;

+ how schools can respond to cyberbullying.

INTRODUCTION

This chapter presents statistics which illustrate that cyberbullying is a prevalent and worrying issue among children and young people. The growth of technology and its popularity have resulted in a variety of forms of bullying, many of which are subtle. Most social media companies have clear policies on online bullying. However, reported abuse is not always addressed and is therefore left unchallenged. This chapter discusses the effects of cyberbullying on victims and highlights ways in which you can respond to this issue.

WHAT IS CYBERBULLYING?

Cyberbullying is bullying which takes place over the internet, including bullying which takes place on social media. It takes a variety of forms, including:

+ posting hurtful comments;

+ posting videos which are targeted directly at a person to cause distress;

+ posting photographs which are designed to cause distress;

+ inciting others to make hurtful comments aimed at a person;

+ sending hurtful text messages using a mobile phone;

+ sending hurtful private messages to a person.

This is not an exhaustive list and forms of cyberbullying are likely to expand as new applications and software are developed. Cyberbullying is fundamentally different to face-to-face bullying in several ways. Firstly, victims cannot escape from it when they are at home because it takes place on mobile phones, tablets and computers. Secondly, the abuse is witnessed by a larger audience; messages are in the public domain and can be repeatedly forwarded. This can result in victims experiencing the abuse on multiple occasions, which results in further psychological distress. Thirdly, the evidence of the abuse is usually permanently stored online, which means that the abuse is not erased. These messages serve as a permanent reminder of the abuse and this can result in abuse being continually experienced by the victim.

Most social network sites have clear anti-bullying policies. However, social media companies have been slow to intervene in cases of abuse and, in many instances, abuse has been left unchallenged. The growth in technology has enabled young people to stay in constant contact with each other. While this can be positive, it can also result in children and young people becoming victims of abuse.

One key question is 'what constitutes abuse?' Have you ever received a text message or an email and interpreted it differently to the person who sent it? Have you sometimes thought that someone was being nasty in a message and been upset by it, only to discover that that was not how the sender intended to make you feel? We interpret the information we receive in text via technology without other cues which are useful in communication, such as body language and tone of voice. Sometimes we may feel that another person is trying to hurt us via a message, but they may not have intended that. The critical point here is that users of technology must be taught to use it responsibly. We should carefully consider how our messages might be perceived by the recipient before we send them and whether there is any potential for causing distress. This is part of being a responsible user of technology. It is critical to the development of digital citizenship that every digital citizen understands how to use technology in a responsible way so as not to cause distress in others. Schools should include this as part of the digital curriculum. The important point to emphasise here it that regardless of whether an individual was intending to cause harm or distress, if the recipient of a message feels that they were being bullied and experiences distress, this constitutes cyberbullying.

Have you ever sent an email to someone which was then forwarded on to others? Or have you sent an email to someone who subsequently replied to you but copied others into the reply? Have you accidentally received a confidential email that was intended for someone else? Have you ever been 'told off' by someone in an email but had others copied into the message? If you have answered 'yes' to these questions, how did this make you feel? If you experienced distress, anxiety or embarrassment, this might constitute cyberbullying. Responsible email use is essential. So that messages cannot be misinterpreted, it is important that forms of electronic communication are clear and concise and do not have the potential to cause harm.

HARASSMENT

Harassment is the act of sending offensive, rude, and insulting messages and being abusive. It includes nasty or humiliating comments on posts, on photos and in chat rooms and making offensive comments on gaming sites. Posting false and malicious things about people on the internet can be classed as harassment.

DENIGRATION

This is when someone may send information about another person that is fake, damaging and untrue. It includes sharing photographs of someone to purposely ridicule them and spreading fake rumours and gossip. This can be on any online site or on apps. It includes purposely altering photographs of others to ridicule and cause distress.

FLAMING

Flaming is when someone purposely uses extreme and offensive language and deliberately gets into online arguments and fights. They do this to deliberately cause distress to others.

IMPERSONATION

Impersonation is when someone hacks into someone's email or social networking account and uses the person's online identity to send or post vicious or embarrassing material to or about others. It also includes making up fake profiles of others.

OUTING AND TRICKERY

This is when someone shares personal information about someone else or tricks someone into revealing secrets and subsequently forwards it to others. They may also do this with private images and videos.

CYBER STALKING

Cyber stalking is the act of repeatedly sending messages that include threats of harm, harassment, intimidating messages, or engaging in other online activities that make a person afraid for their safety. The actions may be illegal depending on what they are doing. Cyberstalking can take place on the internet or via mobile phones. Examples include:

+ silent calls;

+ insulting and threatening texts;

+ abusive verbal messages;

+ cases of stolen identities.

EXCLUSION

This is when others intentionally leave someone out of a group such as group messages, online apps, gaming sites and other online engagement. This is also a form of social bullying and is very common.

SPREADING RUMOURS AND GOSSIP

Online abuse, rumours and gossip can go viral very quickly and be shared by many people within several minutes. It is not uncommon for former close friends or partners to share personal secrets about victims.

THREATENING BEHAVIOUR

Threatening behaviour which is directed at a victim to cause alarm and distress is a criminal offence. Taking screenshots of the evidence and reporting it is one way of challenging this.

HAPPY SLAPPING

This is an incident where a person is assaulted while other people take photographs or videos on their mobile phones. The pictures or videos are then circulated by mobile phone or uploaded on the internet.

GROOMING

Grooming is when someone builds an emotional connection with a child to gain their trust for the purposes of abuse and exploitation. It is conducted by strangers (or new 'friends') and may include:

+ *pressurising someone to do something they do not wish to do;*
+ *making someone take their clothes off;*
+ *pressurising someone to engage in sexual conversations;*
+ *pressurising someone to take naked photographs of themselves;*
+ *making someone engage in sexual activity via the internet.*

Groomers may spend a long time establishing a 'relationship' with the victim by using the following strategies:

+ *pretending to be someone they are not, for example saying they are the same age online;*
+ *offering advice or understanding;*
+ *buying gifts;*
+ *giving the child attention;*
+ *using their professional position or reputation;*
+ *giving compliments;*
+ *taking them on trips, outings or holidays.*

(www.nspcc.org.uk)

It is against the law for anyone under the age of 18 to take, send or redistribute indecent pictures of anyone under the age of 18. Groomers can be male or female and can be of any age.

The Child Exploitation and Online Protection command (CEOP) investigates cases of sexual abuse and grooming on the internet.

INAPPROPRIATE IMAGES

It is very easy to save any pictures of anyone on any site and upload them to the internet. Uploading pictures of someone to cause distress is a form of cyberbullying. This also includes digitally altering pictures to embarrass someone.

BYSTANDER EFFECT

Witnessing cyberbullying and doing nothing about it is not acceptable. Some people are worried about getting involved but victims of bullying need brave witnesses to make a stand. Perpetrators of bullying thrive when they have an audience. Making a stand against what they are doing is a key way to reduce their power. Most sites now operate a reporting facility so that online abuse can be reported and addressed. Bystanders are not innocent. They have a responsibility to report abuse that they witness.

(www.bullying.co.uk)

CRITICAL QUESTIONS

+ Have you experienced cyberbullying?

+ If so, what form(s) did it take?

+ How did it affect you?

SIGNS OF CYBERBULLYING

Signs of cyberbullying include:

+ *low self-esteem;*

+ *withdrawal from family and spending a lot of time alone;*

+ *reluctance to let parents or other family members go anywhere near their technological devices;*

+ *finding excuses to stay away from school or work, including school refusal;*

+ *friends disappearing or being excluded from social events;*

+ *losing weight or changing appearance to try and fit in;*

+ *fresh marks on the skin that could indicate self-harm, and dressing differently such as wearing long-sleeved clothes in the summer to hide any marks;*

+ *a sudden change in behaviour, ie anger, depression, crying, being withdrawn.*

(www.bullying.co.uk)

Signs could also include:

+ *anxiousness;*

+ *clingy behaviour;*

+ *depression;*

+ *aggressive behaviour;*

+ *difficulties sleeping;*

+ *wetting the bed;*

+ *soiled clothes;*

+ *risk-taking behaviour;*

+ *obsessive behaviour, including constantly checking their phone;*

+ *nightmares;*

+ *substance abuse;*

+ *self-harm;*

+ *thoughts about suicide.*

(www.nspcc.org.uk)

THE EFFECTS OF CYBERBULLYING

According to the Royal Society for Public Health (RSPH):

Victims of bullying are more likely to experience low academic perform-ance, depression, anxiety, self-harm, feelings of loneliness and changes in sleeping and eating patterns – all of which could alter the course of a young person's life as they undertake important exams at school or uni-versity and develop personally and socially.

(RSPH, 2017, p 11)

Childhood bullying can have long-lasting and permanent effects. It can lead to diminished confidence and poor self-esteem, and these can have a detrimental effect on academic performance.

● Seven in ten young people have experienced cyberbullying.

● 37 per cent of young people experience cyberbullying on a frequent basis.

● Young people are twice as likely to be bullied on Facebook than on any other social network.

● 91 per cent of young people who reported cyberbullying said that no action was taken.

(RSPH, 2017)

CRITICAL QUESTIONS

+ Why do you think the statistics for cyberbullying are so high?

+ What type of bullying is worse – cyberbullying or traditional face-to-face bullying?

The *Life in 'Likes'* research reported that:

+ Cyberbullying was the most talked about issue in relation to the theme of 'what counts as safety?'

+ Many children said that, when faced with cyberbullies, they knew to ignore the comments and remind themselves that the bully must be 'jealous' or 'insecure'.

+ Many children felt confused about whether a mean comment someone writes to them is real or a joke.

+ Many children were uncomfortable when they saw content that was racist or violent.

(Children's Commissioner, 2018)

CASE STUDY

A primary school revised the computing curriculum to address the advantages and disadvantages of social media. They formed a working group of children from Year 4 to 6 who acted as co-producers of the curriculum. The children were asked to identify the types of social media that they used and the issues they had encountered through using social media. They were also asked to discuss mobile phone use. It was evident that many of the children were using social media despite age restrictions being applied to the various platforms. Many of the children also owned their own mobile phones with internet access. The children were asked to identify issues that were important to them. A key theme which emerged from the working group was how to keep safe online. The themes that were identified for curriculum coverage included: responsible use of text messages; social media platforms; the benefits of social media; the dangers associated with social media; creating privacy settings; recognising cyberbullying and other forms of abuse; how to deal with cyberbullying; reporting abuse; digital resilience; being a responsible digital citizen; and critically engaging with digital content, including fake news.

CRITICAL QUESTIONS

+ What are the advantages of giving children opportunities to co-create the curriculum?

+ Should children in the early years and Key Stage 1 receive lessons on social media?

● 56 per cent of young people said they have seen others be bullied online.

● 42 per cent have felt unsafe online.

● 47 per cent of young people have received nasty profile comments.

● 62 per cent have been sent nasty private messages via smartphone apps.

(www.bullying.co.uk)

Research by Young Minds found that:

+ young people feel that social media has a negative impact on how they feel about themselves;

+ cyberbullying was more prevalent during adolescence;

+ girls were more likely to experience cyberbullying than boys;

+ children aged 11–12 reported the lowest incidents of cyberbullying;

+ children and young people under the age of 25 who become victims of cyberbullying are more than twice as likely to enact self-harm and attempt suicide than non-victims;

+ there are emerging causal links between cyberbullying and children's mental health;

+ the damaging effects of cyberbullying can last into adulthood;

+ adolescents who are bullied are also more likely to misuse alcohol and drugs than those who are not bullied;

+ certain groups of children are more at risk of cyberbullying. These include those with special educational needs and young people who identify as LGBT.

(https://youngminds.org.uk)

CASE STUDY

A secondary school developed a scheme of peer digital mentors. Older students with a high level of digital literacy and digital responsibility were recruited to be digital ambassadors. They assisted with the delivery of aspects of the digital curriculum by leading sessions to younger students on digital literacy, digital citizenship and digital responsibility. They led sessions on how to keep safe online, cyberbullying and responsible and safe use of social media. They planned a student-led conference on social media which was attended by all students in Year 8. They developed a student digital journal on 'digital lives' which they edited and younger students contributed to the content for the journal. Content included poems, stories, reflections, artwork and blogs. The ambassadors were paired with younger students whose digital skills were less developed. They worked with these students individually to help them develop their digital literacy skills and introduced them to applications.

CRITICAL QUESTIONS

+ What are the benefits of peer mentoring?
+ What aspects would teachers need to carefully consider if students are given opportunities to lead workshops?

STRATEGIES FOR ADDRESSING CYBERBULLYING

Schools cannot address cyberbullying in isolation. Social media companies and parents also have a responsibility to address cyberbullying. According to the *Life in 'Likes'* report, social media companies should *'recognise the needs of children under 13 who are using their platforms and incorporate them in service design or do more to address underage use'* (Children's Commissioner, 2018, p 5). Social media companies have a responsibility to:

+ remove accounts of those who are not using social media responsibly;
+ report child abuse to the police;
+ take swift action where abuse is taking place.

In addition, software companies have a responsibility to:

+ design safe products for children by adopting the principle of 'safety first' from the product design stage;
+ create 'walled-garden' products which cannot be infiltrated, and which do not take users away from the product to other sites.

Schools have a responsibility to:

+ provide an age-appropriate digital curriculum;
+ teach children and young people how to be responsible digital citizens;
+ teach them how to keep safe online;
+ teach them digital resilience;
+ teach digital literacy skills so that they can keep themselves safe online;

+ ensure that the curriculum is regularly updated so that it is relevant.

Parents have a responsibility to:

+ provide clear rules about when and where their children can access the internet;

+ establish time limits for internet use;

+ apply filters and blockers to internet-enabled devices;

+ develop their own digital literacy skills so that they can support their child to stay safe online.

Children and young people have responsibilities as digital citizens to:

+ challenge and report abuse when they witness it;

+ treat other people with respect in the digital community;

+ ensure that their accounts are protected by setting privacy settings;

+ report abuse if they are a recipient of it;

+ develop their own digital literacy skills so that they can stay safe in the digital world;

+ develop digital resilience.

CRITICAL QUESTIONS

+ What other stakeholders have a responsibility to keep children and young people safe in the digital world?

+ How can schools support parents with their digital responsibilities?

 18 per cent of young people experienced being unfriended or blocked, but did not see this as a form of cyberbullying.

 63 per cent of children and young people who have experienced online bullying in the last year said they would not tell their parents if something upset them on social media.

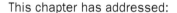

Of those currently experiencing a mental health problem, over two-thirds (68 per cent) said they experienced cyberbullying in the last year, compared to 22 per cent who have no experience of a mental health condition.

(https://youngminds.org.uk)

SUMMARY

This chapter has emphasised the various forms of cyberbullying which children and young people may experience. It has emphasised that cyberbullying can have a detrimental impact on mental health, confidence, self-esteem and academic development. It has highlighted that cyberbullying can have long-lasting effects which last into adulthood. It has addressed the responsibilities of schools, parents, product developers and social media companies in relation to cyberbullying. Forms of cyberbullying will become increasingly sophisticated as technology continues to advance. Schools have a responsibility to keep abreast of developments and ensure that the digital curriculum that is offered to children and young people is relevant and has currency.

CHECKLIST

This chapter has addressed:

✓ different types of cyberbullying;

✓ the effects of cyberbullying on children and young people;

✓ the responsibilities of schools, social media companies, parents and product developers.

FURTHER READING

Campbell, M and Bauman, S (2017) *Reducing Cyberbullying in Schools: International Evidence-Based Best Practices*. Cambridge, MA: Academic Press.

Jones, E (2018) *What's Cyberbullying? (What's the Issue?)* New York: Kidhaven Publishing.

✛ CHAPTER 5

SOCIAL MEDIA AND THE ROLE OF SCHOOLS

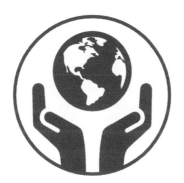

PROFESSIONAL LINKS

This chapter addresses the following:

- Education for a Connected World (UK Council for Child Internet Safety, 2018).

- The Prevent Duty (DfE, 2015).

- Keeping Children Safe in Education: Statutory Guidance for Schools and Colleges (DfE, 2018).

- Teachers' Standards Part 2 (DfE, 2011).

CHAPTER OBJECTIVES

By the end of this chapter you will understand:

+ some of the challenges that social media presents to teachers;

+ some of the opportunities social media can offer to teachers;

+ possible whole school approaches to social media use.

INTRODUCTION

Social media is a rapidly growing and increasingly significant medium within modern culture, with 96 per cent of 16–24 year-olds having some form of social media account (Ofcom, 2017a). This chapter outlines some of the challenges and opportunities that social media presents for staff and pupils within schools and other educational settings.

WHAT IS SOCIAL MEDIA?

Social media is the common term used to refer to a group of services that run as websites, platforms and dedicated apps/services on a range of devices including computers, smartphones and tablets. These services allow users to create, publish and share information in various media formats to communicate with each other.

Social media emerged from the evolution of Web 2.0 technologies which provided opportunities for the perception of technology to change. It has been argued that *'the evolution of the Internet in the Web 2.0 era has been critical in transforming people's attitudes'* (Kevin Yi-Lwern and Yi Long, 2014), leading to the mass proliferation of the 'power to publish'. This represented a shift away from the traditional publishing hierarchy where only large organisations such as news groups and large businesses had the ability to create and share content with the masses. Web 2.0 provided an *'architecture of participation'* (O'Reilly, 2005) that allowed any individual, with access to the internet, to consume content shared by anyone else and equally to publish content that could potentially be seen by, commented on and shared by anyone in the world.

The use of social media has become an integral part of many people's lives, connecting them with friends, family and strangers from across the globe.

(Children's Commissioner, 2018)

This shift, from only consuming media to the ability to create and publish content, has led to a significant shift in the level of individual responsibility that falls to each individual user of these online spaces.

Current popular examples include:

- Facebook – social networking service – 2.19 billion monthly active users worldwide in the first quarter 2018.
- WhatsApp – mobile messaging app – 1.5 billion monthly active users.
- Instagram – mainly mobile photo sharing network – 1 billion monthly active users.
- Twitter – micro-blogging service – 336 million monthly active users worldwide in the first quarter 2018.
- Snapchat – social messaging and photo sharing app – 191 million daily active users worldwide in the first quarter 2018.

(Statistica, 2018a–e)

ADDRESSING ONLINE ABUSE

As with all forms of communication, social media can be used for abuse. Given the huge growth in social media use it is perhaps not surprising that online abuse or cyberbullying is also a growing issue for young people. No longer is this type of activity confined to the playground – mobile technologies enable bullies to potentially affect individuals anywhere, including in the privacy of their own rooms and at any time of the day or night. Conversely, research suggests that 88 per cent of 16–18 year-olds have emotionally supported a friend on social media (Harrison-Evans and Krasodomski-Jones, 2017).

Technological restrictions can go some way to reducing issues like this but it is only when you work collectively that you will start to address the root causes of these issues. Conversations led by trusted professionals who are knowledgeable and experienced in social media are a good first step to establishing a supportive 'community of practice' (Wenger, 1998) within a school. These can be internal or external to the school. In addition, social media and advertising companies also have a responsibility to address some of the issues.

Just over a quarter (26 per cent) of those polled say they have 'bullied or insulted someone else' over social media, with a smaller but not insignificant 15 per cent saying that they have 'joined in with other people to "troll" a celebrity or public figure'.

Our survey found that the vast majority (88 per cent) of 16–18 year-olds polled say they have given emotional support to a friend on social networking sites, and this figure differs little by gender or frequency of social media use.

(Harrison-Evans and Krasodomski-Jones, 2017, p 12)

[A] national survey conducted by Bullying UK found that 91% of young people who reported cyber bullying said that no action was taken.

(#StatusOfMind, Royal Society for Public Health, 2017)

CURRENT SCHOOL APPROACHES TO SOCIAL MEDIA

There is currently a focus in many schools regarding online safeguarding and minimising risk to children by monitoring, filtering and blocking of harmful materials (Harrison-Evans and Krasodomski-Jones, 2017). This aspect of understanding plays an important role in the protection of children online but does have its limitations. For example, if a school chooses to manage access to popular media services on their network, this can only occur during the school day and only while the children are using the school's own network and/or devices. However, personal devices such as smartphones enable children to still access these social media services through the mobile data networks. This results in pupils' online activity being pushed to their own personal devices and via private data networks, making it far less visible to the school.

Blanket bans like this could be seen as akin to denying the existence of roads beyond the school gates, because of their potential to cause harm. For the year ending June 2017, 27,130 people were killed or seriously injured on UK roads (Department for Transport, 2017). Roads have the potential to cause harm. Yet, despite this, all the children, school staff and parents will have likely used, walked across and/or driven down roads to get to school each morning and will be expected to use roads safely as a fundamental part of daily life. Schools teach road safety to minimise risk. Social media is now integral to people's daily lives and therefore schools should respond to risk by teaching internet safety.

Informing the conversation about what is safe and appropriate behaviour on and around roads is provided to help children develop their own understanding of the risks in that environment. Teaching a core set of rules (the 'Green Cross Code') helps each individual to develop this understanding, allowing them to apply this understanding to different scenarios as they may come across them in their lives.

While blanket social media bans can reduce the visibility of issues within the school environment, it can also be argued that approaches such as this create an artificial, sanitised version of the internet that pushes issues somewhere less visible. It is a 'sticking plaster' that fails to address the root causes of inappropriate social media use and also fails to prepare children for the realities of the internet that they will be able to access beyond or even within the school gates.

In addition to this, connected mobile devices are the reality of modern working practices. Not preparing students to use these devices appropriately, effectively, safely and responsibly would be doing them a disservice. It should be a priority for all students to have the opportunity to contribute to these online spaces in a safe and controlled manner. This will help them to develop an understanding of the ethical, moral and emotional elements that influence behaviours here.

This increase in the private use of the internet by young people is likely to hinder attempts to prevent them from encountering online risks such as by restricting their access to inappropriate websites and supervising their online activities. Similarly, the growth in instant messaging means that parents or teachers are often not aware of activity online, such as a conversation in a Whatsapp group as opposed to on a Facebook profile.

(Frith, 2017, p 13)

67

A key shift for many schools will be to acknowledge the realities of pupils' social media use and move from only a 'policing activity' to a more informed modelling role that provides ethical, moral and emotional guidance to inform and empower users of social media.

The legal age for joining most popular social media networks is 13. However, some children create accounts well before this. The structured introduction of responsible use of social media should be achieved through informed education, using case study examples which focus on the human behaviours of these interactions. Such activities can, and often should, take place offline to prompt discussion and reflections on the thoughts, feelings and emotions of both the content creator and content consumers.

Key recommendations are stated below.

Government: Digital literacy in schools. Broaden digital literacy education beyond safety messages, to develop children's critical awareness and resilience and understanding of algorithms, focusing on the transition stage from primary to secondary school.

+ Digital literacy must be applicable to children's everyday experiences so that they are able to apply strong principles in different contexts. For example, the research shows that while children are aware of the message to 'be themselves', when online they often adapt their behaviour in order to gain social approval.

+ Digital literacy should aim to develop children's critical awareness of the imagery presented on social media – by friends, celebrities, brands and others – to enable them to differentiate between curated, often digitally altered, images and people's real lives.

+ Children should be taught about the techniques and algorithms that social media platforms employ to influence what children see online, and to help them understand that they are often designed to prevent children disengaging.

+ Where digital literacy is taught as part of relationships and sex education, children should be taught to recognise the power of peer pressure on social media along with techniques that empower them to switch off and help friends to do the same.

Guidance for parents: Inform parents about the ways in which children's social media use changes with age, particularly on entry to secondary school, and help them support children to use social media in a positive way, and to disengage from it.

Schools: Improve teachers' knowledge about the impacts of social media on children's well-being and encourage peer-to-peer learning.

Social media companies: Recognise the needs of children under 13 who are using their platforms and incorporate them in service design or do more to address underage use.

(Children's Commissioner, 2018)

CRITICAL QUESTIONS

+ As an educator, do you see it as your responsibility to inform discussions around appropriate use of social media?

+ What benefits do see of young people learning to behave appropriately online?

+ Can you be a positive, responsible role model in the social media space?

+ Do you think you should be teaching young people to take personal responsibility for their online actions and the potential consequences of these actions?

+ Should you be informing them about the potential consequences of a positive/negative digital footprint in relation to their relationships with others, employment and the law?

School staff have generally been proactive in responding to emerging risks from online social networking, with over 80 per cent of our survey respondents saying that that they had received some form of guidance at school, but it is unclear how effective much of this guidance is. Our survey results suggest there is no relationship between education and improved online conduct.

(Harrison-Evans and Krasodomski-Jones, 2017, p 15)

- Three-quarters (74 per cent) of 12–15 year-olds have a profile on a social media or messaging site or app. No 3–4 year-olds (0 per cent) and 3 per cent of 5–7 year-olds have a profile, rising to almost a quarter (23 per cent) of 8–11 year-olds. None of these measures have changed since 2016.

- Among those with a social media profile, 12–15 year-olds are less likely than in 2016 to use Facebook (74 per cent vs 82 per cent) and more likely to use WhatsApp (32 per cent vs 24 per cent).

- Less than half (40 per cent) of 12–15 year-olds with a profile say that Facebook is their main social media profile (down from 52 per cent in 2016) while 32 per cent now say that Snapchat is their main profile (up from 16 per cent).

- Three-quarters (76 per cent) of 12–15 year-olds who go online have heard of live streaming services such as Facebook Live, YouTube Live or Instagram Live. One in ten (10 per cent) have personally shared videos using a live streaming service and a third (35 per cent) have not shared content but have watched live streams.

- More than half of all 8–11 year-olds (56 per cent) and 12–15 year-olds (61 per cent) play games online. More than one in ten 8–11 year-olds (13 per cent) and 17 per cent of 12–15 year-olds say they play games online with people they have never met. These measures are unchanged since 2016.

- Among those who play online games, 15 per cent of 8–11 year-olds and 19 per cent of 12–15 year-olds say they use chat features within the game to talk to people they only know through the game, also unchanged since 2016.

(Ofcom, 2017b)

CHALLENGES FOR TEACHERS' ONLINE LIVES

Each member of staff within a school needs to consider their own digital footprint from a moral, ethical and emotional perspective. An individual teacher or pupil may be very technically able and familiar with a specific social network. However, despite their familiarity with digital technology, many often lack information literacy skills (Barnes et al, 2007) and *'the intellectual tools to think critically about much of their experience'* (Alexander, 2008, p 200). This can hamper their ability to make appropriate judgements about the type of materials they are sharing and with whom they are sharing them.

A common issue that arises for teachers is a 'blurring of the boundaries' that can occur when using the same device (often smartphones or tablets) to be active on social media in several different 'roles' (Josefsson et al, 2015). Research also suggests that the judgement applied to online identities varies widely within the education sector. This is often attributed to the education-recruiters applying the potential judgement of parents, board members and other critical groups to content, often resulting in very conservative decision-making (Mitchell, 2018).

Posts from the past or even from old/dormant social media accounts can also cause issues for individuals. Bear in mind that due to instant sharing and the global nature of the internet you should consider that 'the internet doesn't forget' and it is very hard to remove content once it has been posted. However, new laws around the right to be forgotten can make content more difficult to find subject to specific conditions. You can find out more about this from the Information Commissioner's Office website (ico.org.uk).

Much of the guidance for teachers around using social media refers to 'alternative' or 'alias' accounts using fake names. This approach will often breach the terms and conditions of some social media services but more importantly does not address the moral, ethical or emotional impact of the content being shared. These questions should be at the heart of all social media posts from education professionals and play an important role in managing your own online reputation or digital footprint.

In addition, fake accounts are often linked back to real individuals by association and posts on 'private' online chats or messaging boards only remain private throughout the duration that all 'members' co-operate. It is very easy for one member of a group to screen-shot a conversation and make it public. So, consider *what* you say online, not only *where* and *to whom*.

71

Many teachers and professionals use social media sites, such as Facebook, Twitter and WhatsApp, in order to stay in touch with friends and family, to share ideas and get information.

Here are some top tips for protecting your professional reputation online.

+ The best way to find out your online reputation is to search for yourself regularly on a search engine. Use your name and location first and then check variations of your name and even nicknames.

+ Always think before you post. Is that photo appropriate? Could that joke be seen as offensive? Be mindful when sharing pictures or posts or liking content online which could bring your reputation into disrepute.

+ Use privacy settings and safety features which are provided by social media sites to help you manage who can contact you and see the things you share online. The UK Safer Internet Centre provides more detailed information on putting privacy settings in place.

(Childnet International, 2018)

CRITICAL QUESTIONS

Regularly ask yourself the following questions.

+ Do you engage in social media? Do you do so responsibly?

+ Are you aware of your school's policy on staff social media use? Do you agree with it?
   - If not, why not and can you be a force for change?
   - If so, do you comply with it?

+ Do you feel the need to separate your 'work' and 'social' online identities? If so, why, and do these identities cross over?

+ Would you connect with the parent of a child at your school if they requested?

+ Have you checked any old/dormant social media accounts that you may have had in the past?

CASE STUDY

Emily is a 27 year-old primary trained teacher who has recently joined Lawnsgreen Park Primary School as a class teacher. She is single and new to the local area having recently moved into a house nearby. Emily is also a member of an online dating service where she has selected a picture from her last holiday of her in a bikini with a cocktail on a beach as her public profile picture. She has also updated her personal information with her new location to help the service find matches that are nearby.

Several weeks later, Emily receives an automated notification from the dating service saying she has three 'matches' in her area. On further investigation it transpires that one of the matches is from a member of the public within her defined search criteria, another is a teacher at the same school who is known to be going through a divorce and the third is the parent of child who will be coming into Emily's class the following academic year. She has also received an email from her headteacher to say she would like to meet to discuss reports that several Year 6 boys have been sharing an image of her in a bikini between their mobile phones.

CRITICAL QUESTIONS

+ Is Emily within her rights to have a dating profile as a teacher?

+ Are there any considerations/precautions that Emily could take to prevent issues arising?

+ Imagine that you are Emily. What decisions would you make in response to the different messages she has received? Focus on:

  - the message from the school colleague going through a divorce;
  - the message from the parent of a child at the school who may be in your class next year;
  - the discussion with the headteacher about the Year 6 boys who shared the image of you in a bikini with a cocktail.

WHAT CAN SOCIAL MEDIA OFFER TEACHERS?

As many teachers will testify, social media can be an excellent source of teaching tips, advice and CPD opportunities for educators at all levels.

Social media spaces provide opportunities for groups with similar interests or challenges from across the country and the world to share their experiences for others to draw on. These 'communities of practice' (Wenger, 1998) can also act as a support mechanism for colleagues as well as drawing on collective knowledge to suggest solutions to common issues. The Guardian's Teacher Network (www.theguardian.com/teacher-network), TES (www.tes.com), Childnet International (www.childnet.com) and many other organisations provide links for colleagues to get connected and share their experiences, advice and support.

Social media can also be a great medium to engage with parents about homework, school activities, events or news, thus closing the gap between the school and the parents. The senior leadership team should have a clear understanding of the purposes of social media use and provide simple policies and processes which should be explored through effective training to support all staff. Once established, these policies should be regularly reviewed.

While children have internalised messages around 'online safety', they are not always aware of the more subtle impacts that social media use can have on well-being. Teachers should incorporate awareness of this into education about life online.

(Children's Commissioner, *Life in 'Likes'*, 2018)

WORKING IN PARTNERSHIP WITH OTHER AGENCIES

Establishing a broad community of practice to inform the use of social media within your school is vital to information and changing the school's social media culture. In addition to this, it is also beneficial to involve external partner organisations who can act as 'critical friends' for a school's practice. There are many organisations and charities that specialise in this area and can help you broaden a school's view on guidance and support. Here is a list of just some of the organisations which offer support and advice of this kind:

+ CEOP – Child Exploitation and Online Protection command;

+ Thinkuknow;

+ UK's Council for Child Internet Safety (UKCCIS);

+ UK Safer Internet Centre;

+ NSPCC;

+ Childnet;

+ InternetMatters.org;

+ NAACE;

+ local police;

+ South West Grid for Learning;

+ Barclays Life Skills;

+ Microsoft;

+ Kidscape.

CASE STUDY

Sharon is the headteacher of a large secondary school in an inner-city setting. She has just completed a recruitment process to fill two vacant deputy posts that will also form a part of the school leadership team. Due to time pressures, Sharon was permitted to use the national press to advertise these post, at a significant cost.

Sharon complied fully with the local authority's recruitment guidelines and processes throughout. However, a local newspaper is running a headline story on their website and in print suggesting that the school has just appointed a 'religious bigot' into a senior post. There is evidence of potentially racist and homophobic comments on their Twitter account from roughly six years ago.

CRITICAL QUESTIONS

+ In your opinion, who is at fault in this scenario?

+ Should Sharon have done anything to check the digital footprint of applicants, even when the local authority's recruitment guidelines do not include such a check?

+ Do the public have a right to know about the views of individuals who will be working at a high level at a school, even if their views were expressed several years ago?

SOCIAL MEDIA CURRICULUM: WHAT MIGHT IT LOOK LIKE?

A PROGRESSIVE WHOLE SCHOOL APPROACH

School approaches to social media should acknowledge the reality of their use within the setting and be proactive about encouraging positive online behaviour. As Harrison-Evans and Krasodomski-Jones (2017) suggest, this could contribute to a 'digital charter', which was mentioned in the Queen's Speech in June 2017 (HM Government, 2017b), but with more of a focus on the 'social and civic aspects' of a digital identity.

This should, ideally, be a whole school approach where a community of practice (Wenger, 1998) can be established, drawing together individuals who have an interest in this area, but equally those with a fear or concern related to social media. The membership should be refreshed regularly but should include representatives from all areas within the school – including:

+ pupils;

+ parents;

+ teachers;

+ support staff;

+ members of school management;

+ relevant external organisations.

Establishing and agreeing a common 'code of conduct' should be a priority for the group. A simple and easy-to-follow set of guidelines around online behaviours should be introduced to and explored by all members of the school community. These guidelines should use simple language and avoid jargon and technical terms. They should address key risks such as cyberbullying, spending too much time online, inappropriate or harmful content, sharing too much, fake content, body image and other potential risks to mental health and wellbeing (Frith, 2017).

The 'code of conduct' should act as the basis of activities designed to introduce the ideas of 'digital literacy', individual 'digital footprint' and 'digital resilience' to both the students and staff. Use of technology,

76

including social media, should be integrated throughout the curriculum rather than taught as a separate subject. Therefore, these activities should be introduced through changes to existing subject teaching activities rather than being delivered in isolation or as part of ICT or 'e-Safety' sessions. The aim is to empower individuals to think about and take responsibility for the consequences of their actions and to encourage them to be a positive influence on their own 'digital character' and that of others.

Although this group should predominantly be focused on taking positive action to inform and model appropriate social media behaviour, it should also discuss, agree and record how misuse of social media by members of the school body will be dealt with and who is responsible for this. This should take into account the impact on others, potential consequences and relevant statutory guidelines.

Finally, this group should be open and outward-facing, sharing its collective knowledge with the wider school and supporting the embedding of the approaches discussed into teaching practice.

Further advice in relation to this area can be found on the UK's Council for Child Internet Safety (UKCCIS), UK Safer Internet Centre, Thinkuknow and Childnet International websites among many others.

CRITICAL QUESTIONS

+ Does your school engage in social media as an organisation?

+ Have you reviewed your own digital footprint and do you do this on a regular basis?

+ Are staff within your school supported to use social media responsibly?

+ Are children within your school supported to use social media responsibly?

+ What would you do if a parent of a child at your school requested to connect or friend you on social media?

- 91 per cent of 16–24 year-olds use the internet for social networking.

- Social media has been described as more addictive than cigarettes and alcohol.

- Rates of anxiety and depression in young people have risen by 70 per cent in the past 25 years.

- Social media use is linked with increased rates of anxiety, depression and poor sleep.

- Cyberbullying is a growing problem with seven in ten young people saying they have experienced it.

- Social media can improve young people's access to other people's experiences of health and expert health information.

- Those who use social media report being more emotionally supported through their contacts.

(#StatusOfMind, Royal Society for Public Health, 2017)

SUMMARY

Social media is a significant medium for people today and, as such, schools can play a vital role in modelling appropriate and positive behaviour in this space. Both staff and students should develop their ethical, moral and emotional understanding of the content they create and share. A whole school approach to social media use should ensure that staff, children and young people are informed about their use of the social media space, and are more aware of its potential benefits and risks and its potential to impact upon themselves and others.

CHECKLIST

This chapter has addressed that:

✓ schools should acknowledge the realities of social media use to help inform and address it with staff and students;

✓ schools should encourage individuals to develop an ethical, moral and emotional approach to the use of social media;

✓ it is good practice to establish school-wide interest groups in this area and disseminate what you know.

FURTHER READING

Children's Commissioner (2018) *Life in 'Likes': Children's Commissioner Report into Social Media use among 8–12 Year Olds.* [online] Available at: www.childrenscommissioner.gov.uk/wp-content/uploads/2018/01/Childrens-Commissioner-for-England-Life-in-Likes.pdf (accessed 6 July 2018).

Frith, E (2017) *Social Media and Children's Mental Health: A Review of the Evidence.* Education Policy Institute. [online] Available at: https://epi.org.uk/wp-content/uploads/2018/01/Social-Media_Mental-Health_EPI-Report.pdf (accessed 6 July 2018).

Harrison-Evans, P and Krasodomski-Jones, A (2017) *The Moral Web: Youth Character, Ethics and Behaviour on Social Media.* Demos. [online] Available at: www.demos.co.uk/wp-content/uploads/2017/09/DEMJ5689-The-moral-Web-ethics-and-behaviour-on-social-media-170908-WEB-3.pdf (accessed 2 July 2018).

UK Council for Child Internet Safety (2018) *Education for a Connected World.* [online] Available at: https://assets.publishing.service.gov.uk/government/uploads/system/uploads/attachment_data/file/683895/Education_for_a_connected_world_PDF.PDF (accessed 6 July 2018).

✚ CHAPTER 6

SOCIAL MEDIA AND THE ROLE OF PARENTS

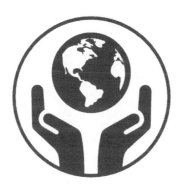

PROFESSIONAL LINKS

This chapter addresses the following:

The Teachers' Standards state that teachers must communicate effectively with parents regarding pupils' achievements and well-being.

CHAPTER OBJECTIVES

By the end of this chapter you will understand:

+ parental use of social media;

+ parents as role models in relation to social media;

+ school–parent partnerships.

INTRODUCTION

This chapter addresses the responsibilities of parents in relation to social media. Many parents did not grow up using social media; they have learned to use social media as adults. Children and young people have experienced their childhoods in the age of the digital revolution. They have never known a world without the internet, without mobile phones and without social media. The internet is an integral part of their lives. It provides access to information and facilitates collaboration. However, it also exposes the younger generation to risks, and parents have a responsibility to keep their children safe, irrespective of whether their digital skills are as well developed as those of their children. Parents are also role models and consequently have a responsibility to model the responsible use of social media. Schools can play a critical role in helping parents to understand more about the risks that children and young people are exposed to in the digital world. Schools can support parents to develop the skills of digital literacy and to understand their responsibilities as digital citizens. This chapter addresses the ways in which schools and parents can work in partnership to keep children and young people safe online.

PARENTAL USE OF SOCIAL MEDIA

Evidence from research suggests that parents use social media to support the process of parenting. They use it to communicate with other parents about parental issues and are likely to use it to communicate with their children as they grow older. Evidence suggests that parents use social media to stay connected and to gain information rather than for entertainment. Facebook is the most common social media platform for parents followed by Twitter, Instagram, LinkedIn and Pinterest.

Parents may be concerned about their child's use of social media. Their concerns may arise because they fear being 'left in the dark' about what their child is doing. They may also be worried about their own limited digital skills compared to the advanced digital skills demonstrated by their child.

CRITICAL QUESTIONS

+ Is it the responsibility of schools to educate parents about social media?
+ How much responsibility do schools have in relation to online abuse which takes place out of school?

WHAT ARE PARENTS WORRIED ABOUT?

Understandably, parents may be anxious about what their child is doing on social media. They may be concerned about their child's safety and may question who their child is communicating with. They may be worried that their child may be experiencing cyberbullying or accessing inappropriate content such as pornography. Some of these fears are genuine concerns. The dangers of the internet and social media are well documented. Many parents have been able to keep a tight rein on their offspring during early childhood. As their child gets older, they naturally seek some independence from their parents. While most parents are happy to provide this, they may be concerned about the lack of control they have over their child's digital life. Most children and adolescents can be trusted to behave responsibly on the internet, but some require further guidance to help them to moderate their online behaviour. It is reasonable for parents to establish time limits for screen time and to restrict the use of technology from private areas such as bedrooms. It is reasonable for parents to apply filters or blockers to restrict access to inappropriate content. However, it is not reasonable for parents to ban their child from using technology or to monitor their child's online activity by checking their phone. Children and young people have a right to privacy and actions like these by parents will lead to resentment.

CRITICAL QUESTIONS

Imagine that you are a parent of a young teenager.

+ You find out that they are accessing pornography online. How will you address this?

+ You discover that your child has uploaded a naked picture of themselves on social media. What would you do next?

+ You realise that they have shared a video on their social media account which shows a friend being cyberbullied. What would you say to them?

+ You notice that they are using offensive language on their social media account. How will you address this?

+ You realise that they are making hurtful comments to another peer in the same year group on their social media account. Who do you need to speak to and what would you say to them?

38 per cent of children felt it was 'very true' that they knew more about the internet than their parents.

86 per cent of UK parents actively mediated their children's internet safety.

67 per cent of parents used restrictive mediation such as time limits or restriction of use of certain applications.

45 per cent of parents used technical solutions to restrict their child's internet use, such as filters or monitoring apps.

58 per cent of children who had smartphones felt that it was 'very true' that they knew more than their parents about using them.

(Mascheroni and Cuman, 2014)

The Net Children Go Mobile study (Mascheroni and Cuman, 2014) found that parents used the following strategies to help keep their children safe online:

+ *Active mediation* involves guiding their child in online safety as well as talking to them about their online activities.

+ *Restrictive mediation* involves creating rules about what children can or cannot do online, installing filters to block harmful content and monitoring a child's online activity by searching their internet history. Additionally, restrictive mediation involves installing monitoring software or checking a child's social network profile.

The research found that restrictive mediation could inhibit the development of the skills needed to handle online risk. Thus, limiting internet access can result in restricting the range of skills that children and young people need to manage internet safety. Research by Przybylski et al (2014) demonstrates that adolescents learn the skills of internet safety through experience. Thus, experience helps them to become more effective at managing online risks.

CRITICAL QUESTIONS

+ Do parents have a right to restrict their child's online activity?

+ Which approach, active mediation or restrictive mediation, do you think is better? Justify your response.

CASE STUDY

A secondary school formed a working group of parents to develop the personal and social education curriculum plan. In response to the question 'what worries you about your child's online activity?' the parents generated lots of ideas. The ideas were grouped together into themes, which formed the basis for part of the Year 8 curriculum. The parents who volunteered to do this also researched the issues and developed a series of workshops. They delivered these workshops to other parents. Themes included practical advice on types of cyberbullying, how to spot it and strategies for addressing cyberbullying as a parent.

PARENTS AS ROLE MODELS

Parents set the tone for their child's use of social media. If parents use social media irresponsibly then children may replicate this behaviour. Parents should model being good digital citizens within the online world. This includes treating others with respect and dignity. Parents should avoid unhealthy online behaviours. These include:

+ making offensive comments which are racist, sexist, homophobic, ageist or disablist;

+ bullying others;

+ uploading photographs, text or videos which will cause distress.

In addition, parents should model the appropriate use of technology by limiting their own screen time and limiting its use when engaging in face-to-face conversation with others. Parents need to establish rules and routines for their child. These might include:

+ banning technology use from bedrooms;

+ turning technology off at specific times, including during sleep;

+ installing internet filters and blockers;

+ not allowing technology use at meal times.

CRITICAL QUESTIONS

You are a teacher in Year 4.

+ A child in your class informs you that their parent has shown them a rude video on Facebook. What do you do next?

+ A child informs you that her parents do not have time to listen to her read because they are always using their mobile phones. What do you do next?

+ A child discloses that their parent has created a Facebook account for them using a pseudonym and that they are using Facebook every day. Who would you speak to and what would you say?

+ A child tells you that their parents never do anything with them or take them anywhere because they are too busy on their mobile phones. What do you do next?

+ A child is upset because his mother has uploaded a photograph of him on social media when he was in the bath. He has asked his mother to remove it but she has refused and it has already been liked by 234 people. His peers in his class have also seen the photograph. What do you do next?

+ Most parents of 5–15 year-olds say they trust their child to use the internet safely.

+ The majority of parents of 5–15 year-olds continue to feel that the benefits of the internet outweigh the risks.

+ One in six parents of 12–15 year-olds feel they don't know enough to help their child manage online risks.

+ Close to half of parents of 5–15 year-olds who go online are concerned about companies collecting information about what their child is doing online.

+ Close to half of parents of 12–15 year-olds whose child goes online are concerned about online bullying.

+ Four in ten parents of 5–15 year-olds are concerned that their child may be giving out personal details to inappropriate people.

+ Around four in ten parents of 5–15 year-olds are concerned about their child seeing content which encourages them to harm themselves.

(Ofcom, 2017b)

SCHOOL–PARENT RELATIONSHIPS IN RELATION TO SOCIAL MEDIA

Establishing effective relationships with parents is essential in order to address the issues associated with social media. It is important that parents do not think you are patronising them and it is critical that they do not perceive that you are telling them how to raise their children. Parents do not like to be judged. They will not respond well if they perceive that the school is blaming them for the problems that their child is experiencing online. They will become resentful if they think they are attending 'parenting classes' or if they perceive that the school is monitoring their parenting skills.

The key to building effective relationships with parents is to demonstrate empathy. They need to feel relaxed, welcome and valued. If you are asked to run parental workshops, you need to build a relationship with parents so that they start to trust you. They need to feel that you are on their side and that you are there to help them. Start off by establishing a sense of 'partnership' by explaining that you are not an expert and that you will learn as much from them as they will from you. Consider posing a few questions and allow them an opportunity to discuss these. Questions might include the following.

+ How does your child use social media?

+ When does your child use social media?

+ How long does your child spend online?

+ Do you know what your child is doing online?

+ Have you established any rules about technology use in the home?

+ What worries you the most about your child's online behaviour?

After you have introduced the questions, allow the discussion to take place between the parents and resist the temptation to dominate the conversation. Ask them to identify the pertinent issues and then develop subsequent workshops to address the themes that they have identified. Consider asking parents to lead some of the workshops. Some parents might prefer a parent to lead the sessions rather than a teacher. However, you can facilitate the discussion.

If you need to report a concern to a parent about their child's use of social media, adopt a non-judgemental approach. Ask the parent if they were aware of the issues and discuss together strategies for addressing the concern. If the child is at risk of harm as a result of their online engagements, explain to the parents who you will refer the case to and what information you will disclose. Reassure the parents that in cases where the child is being abused online by online abusers, that this is not a reflection of their parenting skills and that the priority is to keep the child safe. In cases like these it is extremely unlikely that a child will be removed from their home so it is useful to state this. The priority is to stop the abuser.

If a parent makes a disclosure to you about their child's online activity:

+ listen to them;

+ let them talk and try not to interrupt;

+ make brief notes;

88

+ confirm the record with the parents;

+ explain to them who you will refer the case to and what information will be shared;

+ explain to them what will happen next;

+ thank them for the information and keep in touch with them throughout the process.

If a child or parent discloses information to you about online abuse, speak to the designated safeguarding lead immediately and follow the school's safeguarding policy.

CRITICAL QUESTIONS

+ Do schools have a role to play in advising parents about their own online behaviour?

+ Do schools have a role to play in advising parents about establishing rules about technology use in the home?

According to the EU Kids Online study, parents were slightly more likely to restrict girls' use of the internet than boys (87 per cent compared to 83 per cent) (Hasebrink et al, 2011).

According to Ofcom in 2014:

● 30 per cent of parents were concerned about their child experiencing cyberbullying;

● 26 per cent expressed concerns about who their child may be in contact with online;

● 36 per cent were concerned about their child downloading viruses;

● 21 per cent were concerned that their child might bully others online;

● 22 per cent of parents of 5–15 year-olds were concerned about their child sharing inappropriate or personal photos or videos;

● 25 per cent were worried about their child seeing content which encourages them to harm themselves;

- 25 per cent were concerned about their child sharing their personal details with inappropriate people;

- around one in five parents of 5–15 year-olds whose child plays games were concerned about gaming content (22 per cent) and whom their child might be gaming with through their device (23 per cent);

- two-thirds of parents of 12–15 year-olds who go online (64 per cent) said they had learned about the internet from their child.

(www.ofcom.org.uk)

CASE STUDY

A primary school ran a series of parental workshops which were specifically targeted at parents of children in Key Stage 2. The workshops introduced parents to various forms of cyberbullying and provided them with guidance on how they could help their child to stay safe online. Sessions also focused on the signs of cyberbullying and the dangers of internet grooming. Advice was given to parents on the use of internet filters and they were introduced to a range of applications which children use. Parents were given the opportunity to contribute to the digital curriculum by suggesting themes which should be included.

Our research highlights that (contrary to most of the protection literature) children and young people are active creators of online content. They are generating their own material, posting it online and commenting on posts created on others. This happens equally on public forums (like Twitter and YouTube), closed communities (like Facebook), instant messages services (Snapchat), and has increasingly been popularised through collaborative online games (such as Minecraft or World of Warcraft).

(Young Minds, 2016, p 8)

CRITICAL QUESTIONS

+ Given this research, how can parents intervene when children and young people actively create offensive content?

+ How can schools and parents encourage children and young people to create content in a way which is responsible?

MONITORING SOCIAL MEDIA USE

Some parents monitor their child's use of social media and general internet use. They might do this in a variety of ways, including checking their internet history and installing monitoring devices which enable them to remotely monitor what activities their child has been undertaking online. Parents apply monitoring strategies with the best intentions. They want their child to stay safe online and do not want their child to view inappropriate content. However, monitoring a child's online activity can result in children resenting being 'policed'. It is important for parents to trust their child rather than policing their behaviour. Parents should regularly talk to their children about their use of social media rather than constantly checking on what they are doing. They should introduce reasonable rules in relation to when technology can and cannot be used and the amount of screen time their child should be allowed on a daily basis. However, monitoring their child's devices is a recipe for disaster because the child will resent not being trusted. Establishing internet safety filters is a reasonable step for parents to take but searching through their browsing history is likely to lead to a breakdown of the relationship between a parent and a child.

+ Parents use a combination of approaches to mediate their child's access to and use of online content and services, including: regularly talking to their children about staying safe online, using technical tools, supervising their child, and using rules.

+ Two-fifths of parents of 3–4 year-olds and 5–15 year-olds who have home broadband and whose child goes online use home network-level content filters.

Most parents whose child goes online continue to agree that they trust their child to use the internet safely, and feel they know enough to help their child to manage online risks. They are also more likely to agree than to disagree that the benefits of the internet outweigh the risks.

(Ofcom, 2017b, p 15)

SUMMARY

This chapter has addressed the responsibilities of parents in relation to social media. Statistics presented in this chapter illustrate that parents are concerned about their child's safety online. Some parents respond to this by restricting internet access. However, we have presented research evidence which demonstrates that restricting access to the internet may restrict the development of skills which children need to stay safe online. There is evidence which suggests that adolescents learn the skills of online safety through experience; therefore, restricting their online activity can have a detrimental effect on the development of these skills. We have discussed the importance of parents having regular conversations with their child about their online activity. Parental policing of their child's online activity is unlikely to be effective because children and young people will resent this, and they will find ways to subvert it. Parental mediation of online activity through discussion is likely to be the most effective strategy for parents to adopt to keep their child safe online.

CHECKLIST

This chapter has addressed:

✓ the importance of parental mediation in relation to their child's online activity;

✓ the role of schools in supporting parents' digital literacy skills;

✓ the important role that parents play in modelling digital citizenship to their child;

✓ the important role that parents play in modelling digital citizenship.

FURTHER READING

McCormack, A (2017) *Keeping Your Child Safe on Social Media: Five Easy Steps*. Dublin: Orpen Press.

✛CHAPTER 7

BUILDING DIGITAL RESILIENCE

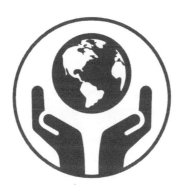

PROFESSIONAL LINKS

This chapter addresses the following:

Schools have a statutory duty to keep children safe and this duty extends beyond the school gates. Part 2 of the Teachers' Standards stipulate the professional duty of teachers to safeguard children and young people.

CHAPTER OBJECTIVES

By the end of this chapter you will understand:

+ what the term 'digital resilience' means;

+ strategies for promoting digital resilience.

INTRODUCTION

This chapter emphasises the importance of supporting children and young people to be digitally resilient. Young people experience multiple risks in the online world and specific groups of people are more at risk than others. Schools and parents cannot prevent children and young people from being exposed to adverse experiences online. However, they can empower children and young people to be resilient when they encounter negative interactions or distressing content online. One way of addressing this is to help young people to critically engage with content online by viewing it through a digital lens. This chapter considers this, along with several other strategies including involving children and young people in developing their own solutions.

WHAT IS DIGITAL RESILIENCE?

Digital resilience is *'the social and emotional literacy and digital competency to positively respond to and deal with any risks they might be exposed to when they are using social media or going online'* (Young Minds, 2016, p 9). Children and young people may frequently be exposed to inappropriate content online, which they find distressing. This includes:

+ sexually explicit content, including pornography;

+ racist, sexist, disablist, ageist or homophobic content;

+ inappropriate language;

+ live streaming of self-harm;

+ violence;

+ content about weight loss;

+ hurtful comments and other content from others, including peers.

In addition, children and young people may be exposed to pop-ups, which include distressing content. They will respond to the content in various ways. Some may be disgusted at the content, others may develop anxiety, stress or depression, and some young people will respond by coming offline altogether. Children and young people who are digitally resilient are able to 'bounce back' from these negative experiences so that they can continue to enjoy the benefits of being part of the digital community.

CRITICAL QUESTIONS

+ What role does digital literacy play in digital resilience?

+ Is online digital resilience as important as resilience in the offline world?

● 12 per cent of young people had experienced 'hurtful or nasty' comments or actions online in the past 12 months.

● 4 per cent had received sexual messages in the past 12 months.

● 7 per cent had seen sexual images on a social networking site in past 12 months.

(Mascheroni and Cuman, 2014)

TYPES OF RISK

Types of risk that children and young people are exposed to online include:

+ *content risks: readily available content on the internet can cause distress;*

+ *contact risks: this relates to a child or young person participating in activities which are adult-initiated;*

+ *conduct risks: these relate to peer-led interactions which include being either a victim or perpetrator of online abuse;*

+ *unmediated social contact: young people are at risk of being exploited or coerced and this risk is heightened due to the anonymity of the internet;*

+ *the potential for mis-reading communication;*

+ *the potential for instantly sharing content.*

(Young Minds, 2016)

According to Young Minds (2016):

+ digital resilience of children and young people plays a vital role in how risks are perceived;

+ one-third of 11–16 year-olds report having been targeted, threatened or humiliated online;

+ children who have greater levels of digital literacy and resilience were better able to mitigate the impact of risks posed by social media and 'bounce back' quicker from difficult online encounters;

+ young people are often acutely aware of the social, moral and ethical dilemmas posed by online communication;

+ young people express a clear sense of proper and improper uses of personal information and disapprove of forwarding content without permission.

(Young Minds, 2016)

WHO IS AT RISK?

Those most at risk of online abuse are stated below.

+ *Children and young people with disabilities are 16 times more likely than their peers to be subjected to persistent bullying.*

+ *Those from minority ethnic groups are more at risk.*

+ *Girls are twice as likely to experience cyberbullying than boys.*

+ *Those in care and those with lower levels of literacy are more at risk of online abuse.*

(Young Minds, 2016)

EMOTIONAL RESILIENCE

We use the term 'emotional resilience' to refer to the ability to control and manage one's emotions in the face of adversity. Children and young people can experience emotional distress as a result of their participation in the digital world. Some manage these emotions well and employ a range of strategies to facilitate this. These include:

+ emotionally distancing themselves from the perpetrator so that they are not affected because the person is no longer significant to them;

+ using specific stress, depression or anxiety management strategies to minimise the effects of abuse;

+ gaining emotional support from others in the face of adversity;

+ refusing to allow others to affect how they feel;

+ viewing the perpetrator as the victim and feeling sorry for them.

Some children and young people have less emotional resilience when they experience adversity. They may be hurt, upset, distressed or angry at what others have said or done to them in the digital world. They might demonstrate less emotional resilience where they have experienced adversity in other parts of their lives. A combination of negative experiences can decrease resilience and 'grind a person down'. Schools have a responsibility to empower children and young people by helping them to recognise that they are in control of their own lives. They need support to help them understand that they may have experienced adversity but through taking positive action, their lives do not necessarily have to play out in this way.

SOCIAL RESILIENCE

We define social resilience as the ability to create and sustain social relationships. When children and young people form strong and lasting social networks in the offline world, they are more able to demonstrate resilience to adverse experiences, including negative experiences in the digital world. Social networks provide children and young people with:

+ emotional support;

+ practical advice on how to deal with negative experiences;

+ social support that helps peers to think about something other than the adverse situation they are experiencing.

From our definition of social resilience, we do not disregard the digital networks that children and young people form online. Digital networks provide support during times of adversity and they can help to develop resilience in individuals. This is particularly evident in situations where young people join networks, which are united by a single cause. The whole network can provide support to an individual who is experiencing a negative interaction, and this can help that individual to be more resilient.

PSYCHOLOGICAL RESILIENCE

Psychological resilience includes psychological constructs such as motivation, confidence, well-being, self-concept, self-esteem, ideal self and intelligence. Children and young people with higher scores in these concepts are better able to cope with adverse experiences. If an individual is motivated to achieve a specific goal in life, they can focus on achieving that goal rather than the effects of the adverse experience. Those who are more confident are more likely to challenge negative interactions online. Individuals with a positive sense of self are less likely to be affected by others because they feel positive about themselves. Schools can play a critical role in improving children and young people's motivation, confidence, sense of self, well-being and intelligence, and by developing these will improve resilience. We now know that these psychological attributes are not fixed within individuals. They are influenced by environmental effects, so they can be developed to empower individuals.

CRITICAL DIGITAL RESILIENCE

Individuals with high levels of critical digital resilience continually question content that they see online. This is addressed in more detail below.

CRITICALLY ENGAGING WITH DIGITAL CONTENT

One of the key aspects of being digitally resilient is the ability to evaluate critically the content that appears on the internet. Children and young people need to be able to identify fake content on the web, which they may find distressing. The internet is full of fake news and other fake content. When they can identify that content is fake, this empowers them to challenge the content rather than to accept it. Children and young people need to develop the skill of critically evaluating content by considering the motivations behind those who have generated the content.

Advertisements, such as those promoting weight-loss products, reflect the financial motivations of the companies that sell the products. It is empowering to understand that content on the web may be under-pinned by economic, social, cultural or political motivations, and when children and young people recognise these influences they are able to question the content that they see.

Children and young people should be empowered to challenge content which is racist, sexist, disablist, ageist or homophobic or content which contravenes any of the protected characteristics in the 2010 Equality Act. They need to be able to recognise content that promotes preju-dice against specific population groups and be given the confidence to challenge it.

Violent content is distressing to see on the internet. Violence is never acceptable and is often exercised by those who are more powerful. The effects of violence on an individual can be long lasting and can result in permanent physical and emotional damage. It is important to teach children and young people to understand how violence affects individ-uals, families and communities. This will help them to critically evaluate violent content.

Sexually explicit content can be distressing, particularly for younger children. Through sex and relationships education, children and young people can be taught to understand that the pornography industry creates nude images and videos that they profit from financially. Themes such as exploitation (of women and men) for financial gain, consent, power and self-respect should be introduced so that young people can critically evaluate content that they see online.

Images that appear online may not be real. Digital editing software is often applied to photographs to completely alter the appearance of the person. This includes:

+ digitally editing an image to make someone look thinner;

+ altering the colour of the skin or hair;

+ making someone's lips appear to be fuller;

+ creating a muscular look to make the body appear toned;

+ altering the colour of the teeth;

+ erasing spots and freckles;

+ altering the size of the nose;

+ altering the definition of the cheekbones.

This is not an exhaustive list but young people should be able to recognise when images have been digitally edited. This will help them to understand that the image they are viewing is not natural. This will enable them to critically evaluate the content that they are exposed to online.

Cyberbullying has been explored earlier in this book. Children and young people should be taught to recognise cyberbullying and to understand how it affects an individual, families and communities. They should be empowered to challenge cyberbullying when they witness it and to report it.

BEHAVIOURAL PROMPTS THAT BUILD RESILIENCE

Technology now has the potential to send messages to individuals to support their well-being. For example, it is possible to receive messages about the length of time that has been spent online to encourage individuals to reduce their screen time. We have already discussed the relationship between social media and mental health. Reducing the length of time spent online will reduce mental health problems and improve well-being. It will also provide individuals with opportunities to form face-to-face social contacts, participate in physical activity and engage in civic participation, all of which are essential for well-being. Reducing screen time will limit exposure to negative experiences online and build resilience to these.

EMPOWERING YOUNG PEOPLE TO TAKE ACTION

Empowering young people to take action in response to inappropriate content is a key aspect of digital resilience. This includes young people:

+ challenging inappropriate content through posting comments;

+ reporting inappropriate content, including abuse;

+ providing online and face-to-face support for victims of cyberbullying;

+ joining networks to support a socially responsible cause.

CASE STUDY

In Year 5, the children explored body image. The teacher asked the class to create a digital scrapbook of photographs they had downloaded from the internet, including social media. The focus of the scrapbook was to highlight ways in which images had been digitally edited. The children annotated the photographs using labels, captions and sentences to highlight the signs of digital editing. They included a range of diverse body types in the book to demonstrate that bodies come in different shapes, sizes and colours.

+ Children's digital literacy is strongly correlated with parental internet use.

+ Increased time spent online means that children and young people are routinely presented with moral and ethical choices.

+ Young people often display a low level of concern about the dangers posed to their safety through internet use.

(Young Minds, 2016)

THE ROLE OF THE SCHOOL CURRICULUM IN BUILDING CHARACTER

The school curriculum should develop a range of positive character traits. These include:

+ moral sensitivity;

+ self-control;

+ empathy;

+ compassion;

+ honesty;

+ civic participation.

Most of these are self-explanatory. Civic participation relates to social responsibility for the local and/or global community. It also relates to social responsibility in the digital community. A good example of this is volunteering within the local community. Children and young people who demonstrate these character traits are less likely to become perpetrators of cyberbullying. Additionally, if young people possess these character traits they are more likely to intervene online when someone is not being treated well.

CRITICAL QUESTIONS

+ What does civic participation look like in the digital world?

+ To what extent is character building simply a way of justifying exposing children and young people to toxic experiences?

DEVELOPING A DIGITAL CURRICULUM

Schools should provide children and young people with a digital curriculum that explores digital risks and strategies for managing these risks. Involving young people in designing the content of this curriculum will empower them and give them a sense of ownership. They live their lives online. They understand the issues and can suggest solutions to address these. The digital curriculum should be age-appropriate and sufficiently flexible to respond to emerging digital challenges experienced by young people.

EMPOWERING YOUNG PEOPLE TO GENERATE SOLUTIONS

Young people generally have a better understanding of the risks they encounter in the online world than adults do. They navigate the online world daily and mediate the risks. One way that schools can build digital resilience in children and young people is to involve them in identifying the risks and empower them by asking them to suggest their own solutions. Too often, the perspectives of children and young people are marginalised by well-meaning adults who think that they know best. However, adult digital literacy skills are often not as well developed as those of young people. Giving children and young people opportunities to suggest solutions to the problems they experience in the digital world provides them with greater ownership of the solutions.

PEER–PEER SUPPORT

Peer–peer support is a valuable way of developing digital resilience. Most young people would rather talk to their peers about the risks they encounter in the online world. They may see this as a private or sensitive topic and might not feel comfortable discussing it with adults. Children and young people can support each other to build the skills of digital resilience. Developing schemes such as digital peer mentors or digital ambassadors is a good strategy for schools to adopt to facilitate peer–peer support. This could involve young people leading workshops on digital resilience with small groups or it might involve matching older young people with those who are younger or digitally less experienced so that they can support peers with the development of digital literacy and digital resilience.

DEVELOPING A MORAL AND ETHICAL CURRICULUM

Schools should provide children and young people with a moral and ethical curriculum that provides opportunities for children and young people to reflect on the ethical and moral considerations associated with online behaviour. If young people do not understand what constitutes moral and ethical behaviour they are not well placed to challenge inappropriate behaviour towards others when they see it online. They are also not well placed to adjust their own online behaviours towards others. The curriculum should empower young people to adopt an ethical and moral stance on specific behaviours and to critically reflect on whether specific online behaviours are appropriate. This could be done through asking children and young people to critically analyse interactions online and to reflect on the motivations of perpetrators of abuse and the impact on victims. They might also be asked to reflect on how they might intervene in online interactions.

DEVELOPING EMOTIONAL LITERACY

To reduce cyberbullying, children and young people need to be emotionally literate. They need to understand how their words or actions might impact detrimentally on others so that they think twice before doing something that could cause distress to others. Schools can develop emotional literacy through exploring case studies of online interactions and engaging young people in discussion of the impact of specific behaviours on others. Younger children need to be introduced to feelings and emotions through personal and social education. By developing emotional literacy, young people are more able to recognise how people's actions can affect others and they can challenge inappropriate behaviour online when they see it. Emotionally literate peers can form a strong network of responsible individuals who are able to challenge online behaviours that cause distress. Schools can adopt a similar approach to that stated above by asking young people to critically analyse online interactions and to consider emotional literacy from the perspective of the perpetrator. They could be asked to consider the emotions of the victim and identify what an emotionally literate response might look like if they intervened in the conversation.

CRITICAL QUESTIONS

+ How much responsibility should schools take for influencing young people's online interactions?

+ Is it better to avoid risk or to confront risk?

+ Is it better for young people who have had a negative experience of being online to come offline so that they are not exposed to risk?

DEVELOPING RESILIENCE IN SIBLINGS OR OTHER FAMILY MEMBERS

Children and young people often support siblings or other family members to develop the skills of digital resilience by supporting them in managing adverse online experiences. Children and young people understand the issues associated with the digital world and are well placed to support each other. Many would not feel happy sharing the issues with parents, but they can provide a source of emotional and practical support for other people in their family. They might intervene in online interactions or provide emotional support when a family member has experienced an adverse situation online. They might also provide practical advice on how their family member can 'manage' the problem.

CRITICAL QUESTIONS

+ Is it helpful to intervene on behalf of others when online behaviours are inappropriate?

+ What are the advantages of intervening in this way?

+ What are the disadvantages?

RISK AVOIDANCE

When a child or young person experiences a negative interaction online, they may experience psychological distress. Some young people avoid repeating the risk of a negative interaction by coming offline. The problem with avoiding risk completely by coming offline is that children and young people do not develop the skills of digital literacy and digital resilience because they are not required to confront risk. Protecting children by 'wrapping them up in cotton wool' will not enable them to manage risks in the offline world and when they encounter these they may not have the emotional, social and psychological resilience to overcome them.

CRITICAL QUESTIONS

+ Can adverse experiences be beneficial?
+ Why is it helpful for children and young people to encounter some risk?
+ Can some risks be positive?
+ When does risk become unhealthy?

Statistics on young people demonstrate that:

● 14 per cent had taken naked and/or semi-naked images of themselves, and 7 per cent had gone on to share the image(s) (Martellozzo et al, 2017);

● 34 per cent had seen hate speech online in the past 12 months (Ofcom, 2016);

● 17 per cent had seen content that discussed 'ways of physically harming or hurting themselves' in the past 12 months (Mascheroni and Cuman, 2014);

● 14 per cent had seen content promoting anorexia (Mascheroni and Cuman, 2014).

PORNOGRAPHY

It is now very easy for young people to access pornography online. Schools respond to this by installing filters and blockers that make it impossible for children and young people to view pornography using school devices. However, young people can still access pornography on their phones. Parents may respond to the threat of pornography by banning the use of technology in private areas of the house or by asking their children not to view pornography. Some parents even threaten their child with various consequences if they view pornography. Despite all of these measures, children and young people always have and always will continue to search for and view pornography. It is not possible, nor desirable, to monitor young people's behaviour all the time.

Younger children experience a range of emotions when viewing pornography, including shock and confusion. Some adolescents may be disturbed by pornography while others view it to learn about sex and to copy what they see. They may use it for sexual gratification. Schools play an important role in developing children's resilience in relation to pornography by helping them to think critically about the content of pornography they have viewed. Although schools cannot show pornography to children and young people, discussions can take place in the classroom that focus on themes such as exploitation, the abuse of power and pornography and the law. These discussions may support young people to become more resilient and reduce the urge to search for it. Young people need to be educated about the risks associated with sending naked pictures and sexual videos of themselves to others (sexting) via the internet or through text messages. This will prevent them from making a mistake that they may regret for the rest of their lives.

+ More boys view online pornography voluntarily than girls.

+ At 11, most children had not seen online pornography.

+ By 15, children were more likely than not to have seen online pornography (65 per cent of 15–16 year-olds reported seeing pornography).

+ Children were as likely to access pornography via a 'pop up' as to search for it deliberately or be shown it by other people.

+ On initial viewing of pornography, young people reported a mixture of emotions, including curiosity, shock and confusion.

+ Shock and confusion reduces on repeated viewing, whether pornography is deliberately sought out, or accidentally viewed.

+ Younger children were less likely to engage with online pornography critically than older children and were more likely to report feeling disturbed by what they have seen.

+ Some older children wanted to try things out they had seen in pornography.

+ A greater proportion of boys wanted to emulate pornography than the proportion of girls.

+ Most young people had not produced naked images of themselves.

+ Some young people had generated naked or semi-naked images of themselves; some of them had shared the images further.

+ Just over half of those who had taken intimate selfies had shared them with others; these are mainly, but not always, people they know.

+ There was limited knowledge of how to remove online images of themselves.

+ Most young people thought pornography was a poor model for consent or safe sex and wanted better sex education covering the impact of pornography.

(Martellozzo et al, 2017)

CASE STUDY

A secondary school enlisted the support of the media department. A group of students in Year 9 were asked to make a film about digital resilience. The young people rose to the challenge. They researched the risks associated with social media and the effects of these risks and strategies for developing digital resilience. They went out onto the street to interview a range of people to collect their perspectives on the topic. Some of these included parents. They spent several weeks making the film. The film was showcased in assembly and launched at a student-led social media conference.

SUMMARY

This chapter has emphasised ways in which the digital world exposes children and young people to multiple risks. We have emphasised that banning the use of technology is not a useful response because this does not allow children and young people to develop the skills of digital resilience. Schools and parents can mitigate risks, but they cannot eliminate them. If technology is banned in the home and mobile phones are banned in school, young people will find ways to subvert this by accessing digital content away from places that are monitored. It is important that children and young people can learn how to address risk when they are confronted with it. Developing their skills in critically evaluating digital content and involving young people in suggesting solutions are powerful ways of empowering them.

CHECKLIST

This chapter has addressed:

✓ the importance of empowering children and young people to critically review digital content;

✓ the need to involve children and young people in identifying the issues and generating the solutions;

✓ the importance of allowing children and young people to access digital content so that they can develop the skills of digital resilience.

FURTHER READING

Young Minds (2016) *Resilience for the Digital World*. Young Minds. [online] Available at: https://youngminds.org.uk/resources/policy/resilience-for-the-digital-world (accessed 18 August 2018).

UK Council for Child Internet Safety (2018) *Education for a Connected World*. [online] Available at: https://assets.publishing.service.gov.uk/government/uploads/system/uploads/attachment_data/file/683895/Education_for_a_connected_world_PDF.PDF (accessed 18 August 2018).

✚ CONCLUSION

KEY MESSAGES

This book has highlighted ways in which social media can have detrimental effects on the mental health of children and young people. It can result in anxiety, depression, sleep deprivation and other types of mental health issues. It has also highlighted the beneficial effects of social media. Children and young people use social media in a variety of ways, including for entertainment, networking and as a source of information. The need for schools to keep abreast of developments and to embrace social media as a valuable source of learning has been emphasised.

The book has emphasised the role of schools in teaching children and young people about digital citizenship, and has highlighted the importance of teaching digital literacy and digital resilience. Schools cannot address all the issues in isolation – parents, social media companies, advertising companies and other industries play a critical role in ensuring that children and young people can stay safe online.

Schools will need to adopt a whole school approach to address the issues associated with social media and mental health. Effective whole school approaches to mental health promote positive well-being and develop mental health literacy in all members of the school community. In summary, the following key aspects need to be given consideration in relation to social media.

LEADERSHIP AND MANAGEMENT

Schools should appoint a member of staff to be responsible for developing digital citizenship, digital literacy and digital resilience. In many schools these aspects will fall under the remit of the computing lead. All staff will need training on the impact of social media use on children and young people's mental health, including the use of social media at subject-specific level. Governors should also be trained in the issues associated with social media and the role of schools in relation to these.

113

SCHOOL ETHOS AND ENVIRONMENT

Key to this strand of the whole school approach is the need for schools to promote a safe environment for all members of the school community. A clear whole school policy on social media use should be developed through consultation with children and young people, parents and school staff. School leaders should foster a culture where technology (including social media) use is viewed as an integral part of learning.

CURRICULUM, TEACHING AND LEARNING

A digital curriculum should be developed which addresses digital resilience, digital citizenship and digital literacy. Children and young people should be taught to use social media responsibly and should be taught about the positive and harmful effects of social media. Schools should ensure that children and young people can critically evaluate content that they see online.

STUDENT VOICE

Schools should involve children and young people in the development of a whole school digital policy and they should be given opportunities to co-construct the digital curriculum. This will ensure that the curriculum addresses topics which they view as important. Additionally, schools should consider developing the role of peer digital champions who can act as peer mentors. The mentors could take responsibility for:

+ leading lessons in the digital curriculum;
+ providing support for younger pupils who have experienced the negative effects of social media;
+ providing mentoring on developing digital literacy skills.

STAFF DEVELOPMENT, HEALTH AND WELL-BEING

All staff in school should be provided with training on how to identify and support pupils with mental health needs. Additionally, school leaders should use technology responsibly by developing clear rules on when staff can and cannot be contacted via technology. Staff may need training on how to integrate social media into subject-specific lessons.

IDENTIFYING NEED AND MONITORING IMPACT

Schools should develop universal approaches to support the identification of mental health needs. Some children and young people may demonstrate visible signs of mental health needs, while others will not. Schools should consider how they will identify children who are developing or have developed mental health needs because of technology use. School-level interventions should be provided to ensure that children and young people receive appropriate support and the impact of these interventions should be monitored.

WORKING WITH PARENTS/CARERS

Parents, carers and the wider family play an important role in influencing children and young people's emotional health and well-being. Schools should provide digital support for parents to enable them to understand the positive and negative effects of social media use on children and young people. Schools should provide digital literacy sessions for parents so that they can help their children to stay safe online. Additionally, schools should help parents to understand their role as digital role models so that parents are able to model appropriate online behaviours to their child.

TARGETED SUPPORT

Delays in identifying and meeting emotional and mental health needs can have detrimental effects on all aspects of children and young people's lives, including their chances of reaching their potential and leading happy and healthy lives as adults. Schools should work collaboratively with other professionals to ensure that children and young people get the support they need.

✚ REFERENCES

Alexander, B and Katz, R N (2008)

Social Networking in Higher Education. In Katz, R N (ed) *The Tower and the Cloud: Higher Education in the Age of Cloud Computing* (pp 197–201). Boulder, CO: Educause.

Barnes, K, Marateo, R C and Ferris, S P (2007)

Teaching and Learning with the Net Generation. *Innovate: Journal of Online Education*, 3(4): 1–8. [online] Available at: https://nsuworks.nova.edu/innovate/vol3/iss4/1 (accessed 17 September 2018).

Boyd, D (2008)

Taken Out of Context: American Teen Sociality in Networked Publics. Berkeley, CA: University of California. [online] Available at: www.danah.org/papers/TakenOutOfContext.pdf (accessed 18 August 2018).

British Youth Council (2017)

Youth Select Committee. British Youth Council.

Childnet International (2018)

Professional Reputation. [online] Available at: www.childnet.com/teachers-and-professionals/for-you-as-a-professional/professional-reputation (accessed 5 July 2018).

Children's Commissioner (2018)

Life in 'Likes': Children's Commissioner Report into Social Media Use among 8–12 Year Olds. [online] Available at: www.childrenscommissioner.gov.uk/wp-content/uploads/2018/01/Childrens-Commissioner-for-England-Life-in-Likes.pdf (accessed 6 July 2018).

Christensen, H, Batterham, P and O'Dea, B (2014)

E-Health Interventions for Suicide Prevention. *International Journal of Environmental Research and Public Health*, 11(8): 8193–212.

DfE (2011)

Teachers' Standards Guidance for School Leaders, School Staff and Governing Bodies. [online] Available at: www.gov.uk/government/publications/teachers-standards (accessed 17 September 2018).

DfE (2015)

The Prevent Duty: Departmental Advice for Schools and Childcare Providers. [online] Available at: www.gov.uk/government/publications/protecting-children-from-radicalisation-the-prevent-duty (accessed 17 September 2018).

DfE (2018)

Keeping Children Safe in Education: Statutory Guidance for Schools and Colleges. [online] Available at: www.gov.uk/government/publications/keeping-children-safe-in-education–2 (accessed 17 September 2018).

Department for Transport (2017)

Reported Road Casualties Great Britain, Provisional Estimates: April to June 2017. [online] Available at: www.gov.uk/government/statistics/reported-road-casualties-great-britain-provisional-estimates-april-to-june-2017 (accessed 5 July 2018).

Frith, E (2017)

Social Media and Children's Mental Health: A Review of the Evidence. Education Policy Institute. [online] Available at: https://epi.org.uk/wp-content/uploads/2018/01/Social-Media_Mental-Health_EPI-Report.pdf (accessed 5 July 2018).

Harrison-Evans, P and Krasodomski-Jones, A (2017)

The Moral Web: Youth Character, Ethics and Behaviour on Social Media. Demos. [online] Available at: www.demos.co.uk/wp-content/uploads/2017/09/DEMJ5689-The-moral-Web-ethics-and-behaviour-on-social-media-170908-WEB-3.pdf (accessed 2 July 2018).

Hasebrink, U, Görzig, A, Haddon, L, Kalmus, V and Livingstone, S (2011)

Patterns of Risk and Safety Online: In-Depth Analyses from the EU Kids Online Survey of 9- to 16-Year-Olds and their Parents in 25 European Countries. [online] Available at: http://eprints.lse.ac.uk/39356/1/Patterns_of_risk_and_safety_online_%28LSERO%29.pdf (accessed 18 August 2018).

HM Government (2017a)

Internet Safety Strategy – Green Paper. London: HM Government.

HM Government (2017b)

Queen's Speech 2017. [online] Available at: www.gov.uk/government/speeches/queens-speech-2017 (accessed 6 July 2018).

Hofmann, W, Vohs, D and Baumeister, R (2012)
What People Desire, Feel Conflicted About, and Try to Resist in Everyday Life. *Psychological Science*, 23(6): 582–8. [online] Available at: http://journals. sagepub.com/doi/full/10.1177/0956797612437426 (accessed 18 August 2018).

Ito, M, Horst, H, Bittanti, M, et al (2008)
Living and Learning with New Media: Summary of Findings from the Digital Youth Project. John D. and Catherine T. MacArthur Foundation Reports on Digital Media and Learning. [online] Available at: http://digitalyouth. ischool.berkeley.edu/files/report/digitalyouth-WhitePaper.pdf (accessed 18 August 2018).

Josefsson, P, Hrastinski, S, Pargman, D, et al (2015)
The Students, the Private and the Professional Role: Students' Social Media Use. *Education Information Technologies*, 21(6): 1583–94.

Kevin Yi-Lwern, Y and Yi Long, T (2014)
Recommendations for Healthcare Educators on e-Professionalism and Student Behavior on Social Networking Sites. *Medicolegal & Bioethics*, 4: 25–36.

Lenhart, A (2015)
Chapter 4: Social Media and Friendships. [online] Available at: www. pewinternet.org/2015/08/06/chapter-4-social-media-and-friendships (accessed 18 August 2018).

Lenhart, A, Smith, A, Anderson, M, Duggan, M and Perrin, A (2015)
Teens, Technology and Friendships. Pew Research Center. [online] Available at: www.pewinternet.org/2015/08/06/teens-technology-and-friendships (accessed 18 August 2018).

Lilley, C, Ball, R and Vernon, H (2014)
The Experiences of 11–16 Year Olds on Social Networking Sites. NSPCC. [online] Available at: www.nspcc.org.uk/globalassets/documents/research-reports/experiences-11-16-year-olds-social-networking-sites-report.pdf (accessed 18 August 2018).

Marchant, A, Hawton, K, Stewart, A, et al (2018)
Correction: A Systematic Review of the Relationship between Internet Use, Self-harm and Suicidal Behaviour in Young People: The Good, the Bad and the

Unknown. *PLOS ONE*, 13(3): e0193937. https://doi.org/10.1371/journal.
pone.0193937.

Martellozzo, E, Monaghan, A, Adler, J R, Davidson, J, Leyva, R and Horvath, M A H (2017)

"…I Wasn't Sure It Was Normal To Watch It": A Quantitative and Qualitative Examination of the Impact of Online Pornography on the Values, Attitudes, Beliefs and Behaviours of Children and Young People, rev edn. NSPCC and the Children's Commissioner for England. [online] Available at: www.nspcc.org.uk/globalassets/documents/research-reports/mdx-nspcc-occ-pornography-report.pdf (accessed 17 July 2018).

Mascheroni, G and Cuman, A (2014)

Net Children Go Mobile: Final Report (with Country Fact Sheets). Deliverables D6.4 and D5.2. Milan: Educatt.

Mitchell, C (2018)

Investigating Attitudes to Social Media Use by Trainee Professionals in Higher Education. MRES dissertation, Leeds Beckett University (unpublished).

Natthakarn, K, Komsan, K, Sirichai, H and Chosita, P (2017)

Association Among Internet Usage, Body Image and Eating Behaviors of Secondary School Students. *Shanghai Archives of Psychiatry*, 29(4): 208–17.

O'Keeffe, G S and Clarke-Pearson, K (2011)

The Impact of Social Media on Children, Adolescents, and Families. *Pediatrics*, 127(4): 800–4.

O'Reilly, T (2005)

Web 2.0: Compact Definition? [online] Available at: http://radar.oreilly.com/2005/10/web-20-compact-definition.html (accessed 2 July 2018).

OECD (2016)

PISA 2015 Results (Volume III): Students' Well-being. [online] Available at: www.oecd.org/education/pisa-2015-results-volume-iii-9789264273856-en.htm (accessed 18 August 2018).

Ofcom (2016)

Children and Parents: Media Use and Attitudes Report. [online] Available at: www.ofcom.org.uk/__data/assets/pdf_file/0034/93976/Children-Parents-Media-Use-Attitudes-Report-2016.pdf (accessed 17 July 2018).

Ofcom (2017a)

Adults' Media Use and Attitudes. [online] Available at: www.ofcom.org.uk/__
data/assets/pdf_file/0020/102755/adults-media-use-attitudes-2017.pdf
(accessed 2 July 2018).

Ofcom (2017b)

Children and Parents: Media Use and Attitudes Report. [online] Available
at: www.ofcom.org.uk/__data/assets/pdf_file/0020/108182/children-
parents-media-use-attitudes-2017.pdf (accessed 6 July 2018).

Office for National Statistics (ONS) (2015)

Measuring National Well-being: Insights into Children's Mental Health and Well-
being. [online] Available at: www.ons.gov.uk/peoplepopulationandcommunity/
wellbeing/articles/measuringnationalwellbeing/2015-10-20 (accessed 18
August 2018).

Office for National Statistics (ONS) (2016)

Internet Access – Households and Individuals: 2016. [online] Available at:
www.ons.gov.uk/peoplepopulationandcommunity/householdcharacteristics/
homeinternetandsocialmediausage/bulletins/internetaccesshouseholdsandin
dividuals/2016 (accessed 18 August 2018).

PISA (2015)

PISA 2015 Results: Students' Well-being, Volume III. OECD. [online] Available
at: www.oecd.org/edu/pisa-2015-results-volume-iii9789264273856-en.htm
(accessed 18 August 2018).

Przybylski, A K, Mishkin, A, Shotbolt, V and Linington, S (2014)

A Shared Responsibility: Building Children's Online Resilience. [online]
Available at: https://parentzone.org.uk/sites/default/files/VM%20
Resilience%20Report.pdf (accessed 18 August 2018).

Przybylski, A, Murayama, K, DeHaan, C and Gladwell, V (2013)

Motivational, Emotional and Behavioural Correlates of Fear of Missing Out.
Computers in Human Behaviour, 29(4): 1841–8. http://doi.org/10.1016/
j.chb.2013.02.014.

Rosen, L D (2011)

Social Networking's Good and Bad Impacts on Kids. American Psychological
Association. [online] Available at: www.apa.org/news/press/releases/2011/
08/social-kids.aspx (accessed 18 August 2018).

Royal Society for Public Health (RSPH) (2017)

#StatusOfMind: Social Media and Young People's Mental Health and Wellbeing. Royal Society for Public Health. [online] Available at: www.rsph.org.uk/uploads/assets/uploaded/62be270a-a55f-4719-ad668c2ec7a74c2a.pdf (accessed 18 August 2018).

Russell, S and Fish, J (2016)

Mental Health in Lesbian, Gay, Bisexual, and Transgender (LGBT) Youth. *Annual Review of Clinical Psychology*, 12: 465–87. doi:10.1146/annurev-clinpsy-021815-093153.

Sampasa-Kanyinga, H and Rosamund, L F (2015)

Frequent Use of Social Networking Sites Is Associated with Poor Psychological Functioning Among Children and Adolescents. *Cyberpsychology, Behavior, and Social Networking*, 18(7): 380–5. doi:10.1089/cyber.2015.0055.

Scott, H, Gardani, M, Biello, S and Woods, H (2016)

Social Media Use, Fear of Missing Out and Sleep Outcomes in Adolescents. [online] Available at: www.researchgate.net/publication/308903222_Social_media_use_fear_of_missing_out_and_sleep_outcomes_in_adolescence (accessed 18 August 2018).

Statistica (2018a)

Number of Daily Active Snapchat Users from 1st Quarter 2014 to 1st Quarter 2018 (in Millions). [online] Available at: www.statista.com/statistics/545967/snapchat-app-dau (accessed 2 July 2018).

Statistica (2018b)

Number of Monthly Active Facebook Users Worldwide as of 1st Quarter 2018 (in Millions). [online] Available at: www.statista.com/statistics/264810/number-of-monthly-active-facebook-users-worldwide (accessed 2 July 2018).

Statistica (2018c)

Number of Monthly Active Instagram Users from January 2013 to June 2018 (in Millions). [online] Available at: www.statista.com/statistics/253577/number-of-monthly-active-instagram-users (accessed 2 July 2018).

Statistica (2018d)

Number of Monthly Active Twitter Users Worldwide from 1st Quarter 2010 to 1st Quarter 2018 (in Millions). [online] Available at: www.statista.com/statistics/282087/number-of-monthly-active-twitter-users (accessed 2 July 2018).

Statistica (2018e)

Number of Monthly Active WhatsApp Users Worldwide from April 2013 to December 2017 (in Millions). [online] Available at: www.statista.com/statistics/260819/number-of-monthly-active-whatsapp-users (accessed 2 July 2018).

Tiggeman, M and Slater, A (2013)

NetTweens: The Internet and Body Image Concerns in Preteenage Girls. *The Journal of Early Adolescence*, 34(5): 606–20. doi:10.1177/0272431613501083.

Wenger, E (1998)

Communities of Practice: Learning, Meaning, and Identity. Cambridge: Cambridge University Press.

Woods, H and Scott, H (2016)

#sleepyteens: Social Media Use in Adolescence is Associated with Poor Sleep Quality, Anxiety, Depression and Low Self-esteem. *Journal of Adolescence*, 51: 41–9. doi:10.1016/j.adolescence.2016.05.008.

Xanidid, N and Brignell, C (2016)

The Association Between the Use of Social Network Sites, Sleep and Cognitive Function During the Day. *Computers in Human Behavior*, 55, Part A: 121–6. [online] Available at: www.sciencedirect.com/science/article/pii/S0747563215301357 (accessed 18 August 2018).

Young Minds (2016)

Research into Children and Young People's Social and Emotional Wellbeing Online. London: Young Minds.

➕ INDEX